The MARS & VENUS
DIET & EXERCISE SOLUTION

Also by John Gray

The MARS & VENUS DIET & EXERCISE SOLUTION

Create the Brain Chemistry of Health,
Happiness, and Lasting Romance

JOHN GRAY, Ph.D.

Foreword by Daniel G. Amen, M.D.

St. Martin's Press ✠ New York

This book is dedicated with deepest love and affection
to my wife, Bonnie Gray.
Her love, vulnerability, wisdom, and commitment
have supported me to be the best I can be
and share with others what we have learned together.

A Note to Readers

As with any health or fitness program, readers are advised to consult a physician before making any major change in diet or exercise routine.

Contents

Acknowledgments

I thank my wife, Bonnie, for sharing the journey of developing this book with me. She has been a tremendous source of insight and inspiration. I thank her for expanding my understanding and ability to honor the female point of view.

I thank our three daughters, Shannon, Juliet, and Lauren, for their continuous love and support. Being their father has been a source of great fulfillment and joy.

I thank my editor, Diane Reverand, for her brilliant feedback, advice, and editorial expertise; Steve Cohen for his vision and encouragement; Melissa Contreras for her dedication, hard work, and editorial assistance; and all the incredible people at St. Martin's Press who turned my manuscript into this book in record time.

I thank my international agent, Linda Michaels, for getting my books published in more than fifty languages. I thank Monique Mallory at the New Agency for her dedication and talent in organizing my busy media schedule.

I thank my staff, Rosalinda Lynch, Michael Najarian, Donna Doiron, Jeff Owens, Melanie LaDue, and Michael James, for their consistent support and hard work in organizing my books, tapes, seminars, radio show, and speaking engagements.

I thank my colleague Dr. Zhi Gang Sha, internationally renowned expert on combining Eastern and Western approaches to physical well-being, for his important insights in developing a healthy mind-body connection.

I thank my many friends and family members for their support and helpful suggestions: Robert Gray, Virginia Gray, Darren and Jackie Stephens, Clifford McGuire, Renee Swisko, Robert and Karen Josephson, Jon Carlson, Pat Love, Helen Drake, Ian and Ellen Coren, Martin and Josie Brown, Malcolm Johns, Richard Levy, Chuck Gray, Ronda Coallier, Mirra Rose, Lee Shapiro, Billy and Robin Clayton, Alex Stephens, and Franklin and Adriana Levinson. I thank the many Mars-Venus counselors and facilitators who continue their work in creating understanding and harmony throughout the world.

I thank the colleagues and experts who aided me during my research: Dr. Daniel G. Amen, John Anderson, Sharon and Tawna Boucher, Cher Camhi, Jack Canfield, Beverly Clark, Darcy Cook, Jim and Kathy Coover, Denny and Vone DePorter, Tony and Randi Escobar, Dr. Salar Farahmand, Dr. Mitzi Gold, Dr. Dennis Harper, Reggie and Andrea Henkart, Dr. William Hitt, Dr. Michael and Helen Joseph, Concepcion Lara, Howard Lehman, Dean Levin, Lauren Luria, Robert McCaslin, Dr. Tom McNeillis, Laura Monahan, Tom Nelson, John Regan, Ron Reid, Andy Rodriquez, Daniel Sam, Gaile Sickel, Scott and Geraldine Strub, Daniel Sun, Dr. Brian Turner, Brian Underwood, Martin Van der Hoeven, Dr. Cynthia Watson, and Dr. Jay Williams. I thank the many people who have attended my Mars-Venus diet and exercise seminars and have shared their personal experiences and concerns. Their enthusiasm with this material has motivated me to write this book.

I thank my parents, Virginia and David Gray, for all their love and support, and Lucille Brixey, who was always like a second mother to me. Although they are no longer here, their love and encouragement continue to surround and bless me.

Foreword

Mars and Venus dieting and exercising together—what a great idea! Yet if they eat the same or do the same exercises, there are likely to be fights and disappointments that send them into orbit, just as when men and women try to communicate or make love without considering male and female differences. In this powerful and accessible new book, John Gray, who brought Mars and Venus gender differences and needs into our culture, honors the differences between the sexes and gives practical, gender-specific solutions for optimizing brain chemistry, diet, exercise, romance, and stress management. He has a genius for taking highly complex scientific material and presenting the information in a simple way, then going on to make practical applications that can change people's lives.

Combining these five realms of health is critical, as each area impacts the others. Brain chemistry affects mood, energy, relationships, and eating behavior. Excessive stress affects brain chemistry, communication skills, and concentration abilities. Relationship problems put us more at risk for depression, stress-related problems, and overeating. Yet the answers for optimal health in each of these areas are not the same for males and females. This is the key element of this book: Males and females need their own solutions to balance brain chemistry.

At the Amen Clinics in Newport Beach and Fairfield, California, we have seen firsthand how abnormal brain chemistry can negatively affect lives, and how optimizing brain function significantly improved those lives. Our clinics treat thousands of patients each year with problems ranging from relationship struggles in couples to learning and behavior problems in children to memory problems in the elderly. One of the primary goals of our work is to balance brain function. Our work is based on a set of simple principles that tie nicely into this book.

- The brain is involved in everything we do. How we think, feel, behave, learn, work, and love stems from the actual moment-by-moment function of the brain.
- When the brain works right, we tend to work right. When the brain does not work right, we have significant trouble being our best.
- The brain is the most complicated organ in the universe. It is estimated that we have 100 billion neurons and that each neuron connects to other neurons by hundreds or even thousands of individual connections. It is estimated that we have more connections in our brain than there are stars in the universe. The brain is also the primary user of energy in the body. Even though it is only about 2 percent of the body's weight, the brain uses about 20 percent of the calories we consume.
- The brain is soft, much like the consistency of soft butter, and it is housed in a hard skull that has many ridges. Mild traumatic brain injuries can damage the brain and change lives, yet few people know this fact.
- Psychiatrists and mental health professionals should be looking at how the brain works in people who struggle with learning, behavior, or emotional problems. Looking at brain function provides us with much important information. We have tools available to us today to look at brain function.

- Certain areas of the brain are primarily responsible for certain functions. For example, the prefrontal cortex is involved with concentration, forethought, judgment, impulse control, and decision making; the temporal lobes house memory, mood stability, and temper control; and the anterior cingulate gyrus helps in shifting attention and cognitive flexibility. Problems in each area of the brain—whether from genetic factors, brain trauma, toxic exposure (drug or alcohol abuse), or stress—lead to corresponding problems with the functions of each area.

- Protecting and optimizing brain function is essential in helping people to be the best they can be. In our culture, despite many advances in neuroscience, we act as if we do not understand the brain's immense importance in our day-to-day lives. And we do not honor the brain. For example, we allow children to hit soccer balls with their heads, snowboard without helmets, and never give a second thought to "minor" brain injuries.

- There are many ways to optimize brain function, including the use of supplements, vitamins, and medications; proper diet and exercise; decreases in stress (stress hormones damage brain function); and enhancement of relationships.

One of the most unique aspects of the work at the Amen Clinics is our use of brain SPECT (single photon emission computed tomography) imaging in helping us understand people who struggle with emotional, behavioral, or learning problems. Brain SPECT imaging is a nuclear medicine procedure that uses radioisotopes to look at a living, working brain. SPECT is easy to understand. It shows three things: areas of the brain that work well, areas of the brain that work too hard, and areas of the brain that do not work hard enough. SPECT can see healthy brain function. It can also see the damage from substance abuse or brain injury, the precedents to dementia, and the many faces of anxiety, depression, and attentional problems. We can see physical brain problems in illnesses that were until recently thought to be psychological in nature, such as anxiety or depression.

During the past twelve years, my clinics have amassed the world's largest database of brain imaging studies related to behavior, now over 16,000 scans. We have many before and after SPECT scans that help us know which treatments help brain function, which treatments are ineffective, and which treatments seem to make things both better and worse at the same time. For example, such commonly prescribed antidepressants called selective serotonin reuptake inhibitors (SSRIs) as Prozac, Zoloft, and Paxil, tend to calm the overactive emotional areas of the brain associated with depression, but they also can decrease activity in the prefrontal cortex and give people concentration and motivational problems.

One of the surprising early findings of our work is that you have to tailor treatments to individual needs. Not all people who are depressed respond to the same treatment. Traditional antianxiety supplements or medications work for some people but not others. Treatments need to be individualized, based on gender, temperament, and individual differences in brain function. This was the main reason I was so pleased to write the foreword for John Gray's new book. He takes a balanced, forward-thinking approach that includes a wide variety of ways to optimize brain function, and ultimately relationship and life function.

In our clinics, as in this book, we recommend a wide variety of treatments to optimize brain and life function. Many supplements work by balancing brain function.

We also recommend dietary changes, as John Gray does in this book. Food is medicine. All of us know this intuitively. If you eat the right things in the morning, at lunch, or for dinner, you feel good. If you eat the wrong things, you feel bloated, unfocused, and bad. What if you have three doughnuts in the morning? How do you feel thirty minutes later? Most people feel tired and lethargic. But what if you ate a healthy breakfast?

Your energy is likely to be much higher, and your mind much clearer.

Exercise works through many different mechanisms in the body. Studies have shown that exercise boosts blood flow to the brain, enhancing cognitive abilities, even in the elderly. Exercise also increases serotonin availability in the brain. Serotonin is one of the major mood neurotransmitters in the brain and helps us be flexible and happy.

Romance and relationships are also critical to brain health. In a landmark study on interpersonal psychotherapy (IPT), which teaches people how to improve their relationships, the benefits go all the way to the brain. Brain SPECT studies showed that the function of brain areas critical to mood regulation can return to normal after a short course of IPT. "We're starting to see some fascinating consistency in the data," said Dr. Stephen D. Martin of the University of Durham in Sunderland, England. Researchers at the university's Cherry Knowle Hospital performed SPECT studies on twenty-seven adult patients with major depression. The investigators then randomly assigned fourteen of the patients to receive an antidepressant, while thirteen other patients began weekly one-hour IPT sessions. After six weeks of treatment, both groups had significantly improved scores related to depression. A second round of SPECT studies after treatment in both groups also showed significant improvement, especially in the emotional areas of the brain, indicating patients were less depressed and less focused on bad feelings. The imaging findings, according to Dr. Martin, support the notion that brain changes contribute significantly to both the development and the resolution of depression. Our day-to-day interactions with others enhance or hurt how the brain works. Being more connected to the people in your life helps heal the brain. Love is as powerful as drugs, and usually a lot more fun.

Stress management also helps protect the brain. Exposure to stress hormones has recently been shown to disrupt cells in one of the major memory centers of the brain, the hippocampus. The more stress one is under, the worse one's memory and temper. Learning new ways to deal with stress and overcome it are critical to brain health.

This book has much to teach those in search of a happy, holistic life. A better brain and a better life are now within our reach.

—Daniel G. Amen, M.D., author of
Change Your Brain, Change Your Life

The MARS & VENUS
DIET & EXERCISE SOLUTION

1

THE MARS AND VENUS DIET AND EXERCISE SOLUTION

America is in a health crisis—mental, emotional, and physical. Every day we hear more bad news, not just in our own lives, but everywhere. We are bombarded with terrible messages: one in five boys is diagnosed with attention deficit/hyperactivity disorder (ADHD); teen suicides, violence, and drug abuse have skyrocketed; one out of every two new marriages ends in divorce; one out of every two men over fifty will suffer prostate problems; one out of every three women will endure cancer; 65 percent of our population is overweight; millions of women are clinically depressed, depending on psychoactive drugs to get out of bed in the morning; and millions of men depend on prescription drugs to perform sexually in bed. Enough! The list just goes on and on. You don't need this book to remind you of these facts.

The Mars and Venus Diet and Exercise Solution provides practical and easy answers for the whole list. The book is entitled *The Mars and Venus Diet and Exercise Solution* because it addresses the unique needs of men and women. It is amazing that with all the hundreds of diet and exercise books, self-help books, and psychology manuals available, no one has pointed out how men and women react differently to food and exercise. A general one-size-fits-all unisex solution is suggested without reference to the facts about gender.

HOW FOOD AND EXERCISE
AFFECT MEN AND WOMEN DIFFERENTLY

Let's look at some issues I'll explore in these pages that are not commonly known or expressed in other books and programs:

- Do you know that the same diet plan may cause a woman to gain weight, while a man will lose weight?
- Do you know that a man's diet—not how much he has worked—is primarily responsible for fatigue at the end of his workday?
- Do you know that a woman's diet can contribute more significantly to her feelings of fulfillment than the behavior of her partner?
- Do you know why women require more cuddling and affection and men require more sex to experience healthy brain chemistry?
- Do you know why more men and fewer women experience addictive tendencies to harmful substances, work, or exercise?
- Do you know that more men have the symptoms of low dopamine while more women have the symptoms of low serotonin?
- Do you know that 90 percent of the people who seek counseling are women, and that most demonstrate the symptoms of low serotonin?
- Do you know that 90 percent of the people in jail are men and that most demonstrate the symptoms of low dopamine?
- Do you know why women are more prone to depression than men?
- Do you know why an exercise program to assist a man in losing weight might inhibit weight loss in a woman as well as produce food cravings?
- Do you know why certain food combinations will put a man to sleep but put a woman in the mood or vice versa?

- Do you know that starting a new diet program, even if it is not good for you, will cause a man, but not a woman, to lose weight temporarily?
- Do you know that skipping breakfast in the morning will contribute to depression and cause weight gain for a woman but may create an endorphin high for a man, to be followed by low energy and overeating at the end of the workday?
- Do you know that depression in men has completely different symptoms and different solutions from depression in women?
- Do you know that exercise in general is not good for obese women to begin losing weight, but is absolutely essential for obese men?

Throughout *The Mars and Venus Diet and Exercise Solution* you will gain insight into these gender differences, as well as many more. You will be exposed to cutting-edge research that is not available to you elsewhere. Finally, you will be able to make sense of your health, happiness, and romance without being confused by the myriad conflicting points of view presented by books, research studies, the media, and different authorities.

My goal is to introduce you to basic information about nutrition, exercise, brain chemistry, sex hormones, and stress management. Once you have all the pieces of the puzzle in front of you, they will all fit neatly together, and you will realize why diets, exercise programs, or relationships may have failed in the past as well as why these new insights work. Regardless of past regrets, you will be motivated to try again and succeed this time by creating the neurochemistry of health, happiness, and lasting romance.

PUTTING ALL THE PIECES TOGETHER

While researching this topic during the past ten years since I wrote *Men Are from Mars, Women Are from Venus,* I have asked the question "How do diet and exercise affect men and women differently?" Most of the time, experts I have interviewed don't have a ready answer. As I have continued to ask more questions, consulting with many experts and reviewing thousands of research papers, along with years of experimenting on my own, the various elements started to come together.

This new program is based on modern medical research combined with ancient knowledge. In some ways, you will know more than most researchers. The experts specialize. They have a particular agenda and specialize in accomplishing just that. They are so focused on their own specific area that they are often not aware of what's going on in other fields. For more than thirty years, I have gleaned the revolutionary information contained in this book from specialists in five different areas of interest: brain chemistry, diet, exercise, romance, and stress management.

From distinguished brain experts, I have gathered cutting-edge information based on their research on the chemistry of the brain, research directed at helping the mentally ill. Practical insights derived from this specialized research can affect all areas of your life. Many people display certain mild symptoms that mirror the more severe symptoms of the mentally disturbed.

Most people today display certain mild symptoms
that mirror the more severe symptoms of the
mentally disturbed.

Although many millions of Americans have been diagnosed with mental illness and require psychoactive drugs, it is my experience and that of many researchers that these people are just suffering from nutritional deficiency as opposed to actual brain damage or some genetic defect. Once the brain is fed the proper food through supplementation with amino acids, the symptoms of mental illness begin to disappear, sometimes in just days.

These brain researchers, however, know very little about the issues of healthy, loving couples seeking to have lasting romance, or about the millions of people who are mildly depressed seeking help to find that extra something missing in their lives. Yet the same imbalance of neurotransmitters associated with the different aspects of mental illness also applies to most of the "normal neurosis" that I have observed as a counselor.

Cutting-edge brain researchers know little about applying their ideas to healing "normal neurosis."

Many therapists, counselors, and teachers are experts in the day-to-day concerns of stress management, but they are not experts in weight management, health, or diet. They are not aware of how nutrition affects our mental health, which in turn affects weight gain or loss. Many teachers and programs are teaching relaxation techniques and meditation but may not be familiar with how exercise and diet contribute to our state of mind as well as to our ability to cope with stress.

As counselors begin using this all-inclusive program to assist clients with depression and anxiety disorders as well as relationship problems, the road to recovery will become newly paved. I have discovered as a marriage counselor that most problems couples experience can be resolved by educating them about the differences between men and women. Once we begin to understand, accept, and respect our partner's style of communication, we can be more successful in giving and receiving love. Yet even with these essential insights, without a healthy diet and exercise program to support balanced brain chemistry, many men and women just don't have the energy or peace of mind to put into practice what seemed so easy at the beginning of a relationship.

Too often, people join a Twelve Step program and succeed in giving up an alcohol, drug, or relationship addiction only to replace it with a coffee, smoking, or sugar addiction. Though giving up the original addiction is certainly a positive step, they will still suffer from the stress and distress associated with any addictive behavior until they balance the chemicals in their brains. Emotional healing or recovery is never complete until we balance brain chemistry with appropriate exercise and balanced diet. Any and all addictive behaviors are symptoms of brain imbalance.

Too often, people join a Twelve Step program and succeed in giving up one addiction only to replace it with another.

Current research about diet is brilliantly expressed in many conflicting diet-book bestsellers. Though many diet experts offer their own effective plans for losing weight, they often do not make the connection to the ways brain chemistry or communication skills and romance affect our eating habits. As a result, many of their suggestions work temporarily, but if people are not eating to balance brain chemistry or communicating in ways to stimulate certain hormones, staying on a healthy diet can be nearly impossible.

Current diet plans say little about stimulating the correct brain chemicals to achieve optimum health and weight management.

Though exercise experts have a lot to contribute, many are not yet aware of how different types of exercise affect brain chemistry. Some personal trainers push their clients too hard, only to lose these clients when they give up and quit.

I have put together for you an accessible body of information and insight that is not only easy to understand but effortless to adapt to any lifestyle. My program is not designed to replace what might be working for you already. Instead, consider *The*

Mars and Venus Diet and Exercise Solution as an easy-to-apply routine to enrich the programs you are already enjoying. You will benefit from the latest proven research in the following fields:

1. Diet, nutrition, and weight management
2. Essential physical exercises for stimulating the lymph system, endocrine system, and cerebral spinal fluid and brain system, and for toning your muscles while stimulating the metabolism
3. Brain chemistry for mental health and happiness
4. Relationship, communication, and romantic issues that affect both hormonal balance and brain chemistry balance
5. Stress and mood management for a longer, healthier, and happier life

Studying each of these fields over the last thirty years with particular emphasis on the health and nutrition aspects during the last ten years has led me to create *The Mars and Venus Diet and Exercise Solution*. While many of the insights and tools have taken me thirty years to test and develop with thousands of clients, it was not until 2002 that the whole picture became clear with the added understanding of activated amino acid supplementation for establishing the correct brain balance. With this newly discovered piece of the puzzle, the benefits of all the other proven techniques exploded exponentially.

Millions of people have benefited from my books, tapes, and seminars. With the addition of balanced brain chemistry, those benefits are greatly enhanced and are more easily sustained. Both men and women will benefit even more from my relationship insights. At the same time, parents will more easily apply the many useful insights contained in my book *Children Are from Heaven*. Whether you use my suggested parenting techniques or not, any parenting system works better when your children are not suffering from the brain imbalances responsible for ADD, ADHD, and OCD. With crucial information from each of the five fields of expertise, you will have the basics to understand simple and effective ways of improving not only your relationship with others, but also your relationship with your body.

NINETY PERCENT EFFECTIVE!

You don't have to dedicate yourself to a long, difficult dietary and exercise regime only to find out months or years later that you are not only more depressed but sick as well. These ideas are easy to apply and yield quick results. Most of the time they work right away.

Within days of beginning, you will know if this program is going to work for you. If you don't see results within a few weeks, your condition is not just the result of nutritional deficiency. If you have had a concussion or accident, if your liver is overly toxic, or if you are taking a lot of medications, you may need more time to experience the full benefits of the program. In such cases, other kinds of support are required as well. We will explore these other healing options in Chapter 13 of this book.

My experience while teaching this new program has been that it works immediately for more than 90 percent of the people who try it. I know it sounds too good to be true; I know some of you may be thinking that it can't be that easy. But it is. I have seen it with my own eyes and continue to hear about it every day. While most people are bombarded with discouraging messages and statistics from the media each day, I receive hundreds of messages of immediate and positive transformation and healing. That is why I am so optimistic.

The program is so easy to apply that almost everyone who tries it benefits immediately. Thousands of people have already begun this new program and are enjoying better health, increased happiness, and lasting romance. Many, under the supervision of their doctors, have gradually gone off such psychoactive medications as Prozac. Thousands of overweight people have lost and kept off their extra weight in just a few weeks. Loving couples who had lost some of the initial passion over their years together are now experiencing a renewed and lasting romantic glow. Every day I hear the stories of increased health, energy, successful weight management, and better sleep at night.

In a week you will begin to see dramatic results. Each day I am amazed by how quickly these simple changes create positive benefits. I know some of you may be thinking, "How could it be so simple?"

HOW COULD IT BE THIS EASY?

The answer to this question is simple. Never in history have we had so much wisdom and information available to us, and yet never have we been so confused. In this sense, we are living in a paradoxical time. Every year thousands of books and research studies are published with the latest information to make our lives better. With this information, our lives get better and worse. All of this dramatic change has prepared the foundation for the answers in this book to change your life. Yet the changes that have occurred in our society in the last thirty years are more than a foundation; they are the whole house. Everything you need is available in this house. The only problem is, we don't have a key to get in.

You will find the key to that house in this book. The actual house has already been built and is already available. The foundation is in place. All the research has been done, and all the expertise and support is available. But without the key to using that support correctly, all this is of little value.

Certainly, regular checkups with your doctor and regular exercise will benefit your health, but without the information in this book, people still get sicker as they get older!

Certainly, finding a good job and making lots of money will make you happy, but without the information in this book, work opportunities just make most people tired, anxious, stressed, or overwhelmed.

Certainly, finding the love of your life and taking classes or reading helpful books on improving your ability to communicate will help you find lasting romance, but for most people, the romance will fade without the information in this book.

Getting dramatic results is easy, because there is already so much support available. It is just not being fully utilized. New medical breakthroughs and discoveries are published every week; stores specializing in healthy foods and supplements are popping up everywhere; thousands of new self-help books are published every year; gyms and yoga studios are available in every community; and new and old spiritual institutions are experiencing a resurgence in community participation. What, then, is the magic key to make use of all this potential?

THE MAGIC KEY

The magic key is waiting for you at your local health food store, general nutrition center, and grocery. That's right, it is what you eat that determines your health, happiness, and love life. When you put all the pieces of the puzzle together, what is missing for everyone is just one piece. That piece is nutrition and exercise.

The magic key to health, happiness, and romance is waiting for you in your local health food store and/or grocery store.

Once I discovered the symptoms of nutritional deficiency and an imbalance in brain chemistry, I realized that every person I have ever met, counseled, or read about fits the description. In my career, I have met, counseled, or talked with in my seminars more than a million people. When I say *everyone* can benefit from this message, I literally mean everyone, and I am not making a wild claim. I can't claim that everyone will get the same benefits, because everyone's response is different.

> Having learned to recognize the behavioral
> symptoms of nutritional deficiency, I now
> recognize that everyone I have ever met or
> worked with fits the description.

In addition to nutritional deficiency, some people suffer from brain trauma, birth defects, or the results of extreme abuse of the body from drugs, nutritional deficiency, or the side effects of modern medicine. These conditions may inhibit some of the immediate benefits of the program.

Even for the 10 percent who don't benefit immediately, if the principles of *The Mars and Venus Diet and Exercise Solution* are applied consistently, different degrees of benefits are still possible when coupled with other forms of healing. Depending on a person's preference and condition, there are many effective healing modalities. More and more, modern doctors and therapists are recognizing and even recommending complementary forms of healing involving chiropractors, naturopathic doctors and nutritionists, homeopathy, traditional Chinese medicine, intravenous ozone therapy (legal in Germany but not yet in the United States), intravenous amino acid supplementation, prolo therapy, vitamin supplements, acupuncture, herbs, aromatherapy, energy healing, spiritual healing, chi kung, tai chi, yoga, meditation, positive visualization, and journaling.

By adding the Mars and Venus Solution, those with more serious problems who don't get results right away can enjoy new hope. Each of the above healing treatments is dramatically enriched when patients supplement their healing program with *The Mars and Venus Diet and Exercise Solution*.

As you can probably tell, I am very happy to share this information with you, because I know you too will benefit in a variety of ways. Exploring these five different fields of expertise has been an exciting journey for me, and I know it will be just as exciting for you.

2

DISCOVERING THE
MARS AND VENUS SOLUTION

Ten years ago, when I turned forty, I began to experience that my health was no longer a given. Although I took good care of myself, health and weight management had never been a major concern in my earlier years. After a small skiing accident, I discovered that around forty, the body doesn't bounce back the way it used to. All I did was fall down, and it took six months before I could fully cross my legs in a relaxed manner.

After forty, good health is not automatic.

It was a clear wake-up call: Unless I actively worked to improve my physical condition, it was going to go downhill. This insight is similar to a truth I had already learned about romance and relationships. In the first three years of a relationship, you get free romantic hormones. After that, unless you have good communication and make time to create romance, the passion begins to fade away. You can't expect romance to happen automatically as it did in the beginning. You can create romance, but it is not automatic.

The same is true regarding our health, vitality, and flexibility. For the first forty years of life, health is somewhat of a given, but after that, unless you actively promote good health, your level of vitality decreases and the aging process begins.

**In a relationship, you get about three years
of free romantic hormones.**

I listened to my wake-up call. Throughout my forties, I explored a variety of self-care modalities. I revisited the yoga and meditation techniques I had diligently practiced and taught in my twenties. In those days, I had turned to yoga to develop my mental and spiritual potential, but now I was doing it to stay fit and healthy.

Like many people my age, I began reading and studying all the bestselling diet, health, and exercise programs. I tried many of them, and they all worked . . . at least for a while. Even with my growing expertise, I would go on a great diet for several months, trying to eat in a perfect manner, and then eventually I would swing the other way. I would lose weight and then gain it back. Something was still missing for me.

In a variety of ways, I had the answers, but I was inconsistent. I would exercise regularly for a while, feel great, and then just stop. I would be dynamic at my talks, and then exhausted when I got home. I would be especially warm and friendly to my wife when I was in a romantic mood, but the next day I would be less attentive.

**I would be dynamic at my talks,
and then exhausted when I got home.**

To make matters worse, I thought this degree of up and down, back and forth was normal. I didn't realize there was a problem. Since these symptoms are so common and since I was basically happy, healthy, and successful in life, I had no notion of how much easier my life could be. A little weight gain, muscle tension, low energy, minor joint pain, memory lapses—these were all supposedly a part of getting old. I accepted these symptoms as normal because I didn't know what I was missing!

This ignorance and passivity are rampant in our society. Millions of people think it is normal to suffer the sicknesses of premature aging and regularly take medications as a routine part of their life. Medication should be for emergencies, not a way of life. This is a problem that can be solved, but first you must recognize that there *is* a problem.

Millions of people mistakenly think it is normal to suffer the sicknesses of premature aging.

When the solution to this problem appeared, it took me by complete surprise.

MY TRIP TO MEXICO

For more than thirty years, I have practiced and taught yoga, meditation, psychology, diet, and other mental and physical self-help exercises. With all that, I still had not found a way to *sustain* vibrant health, happiness, and romance. Sure, I was reasonably successful in each of these areas, but the good results I experienced were not even close to what I experience now.

The insight that helped me discover *The Mars and Venus Diet and Exercise Solution* was understanding the power of creating healthy brain chemistry. I knew its application for the mentally ill, but had no idea how balancing brain chemistry could have an impact on the lives of all people. This important journey began during a one-week trip to a medical clinic in Tijuana, Mexico.

A good friend had told me about Dr. William Hitt, a brilliant seventy-six-year-old Nobel Prize–winning American medical doctor and researcher who provides remarkable treatment for people who suffer from allergies and asthma. In one week of treatment, symptoms are reported to vanish, and after a few weeks, to a great extent they are gone forever! This appealed to me. I have had hay fever and allergies to cats, dust, and mold throughout my whole life. With a "perfect diet" and self-healing exercises, I had even learned to heal them and be free of symptoms. To stay allergy-free, I had to continue to eat that perfect diet: absolutely no dairy, no sugar, no bread, no processed food, and no hydrogenated fat. This diet was restrictive to the extreme. The thought of being allergy-free and able to enjoy a variety of foods was attractive, so I went to Mexico to give it a try.

A perfect diet with absolutely no dairy, no sugar, no bread, no processed food, and no hydrogenated fat is not fun, nor is it necessary for good health.

Avoiding the misery of allergies was a prime motivator for me to follow that perfect diet. The secondary result was that I always lost weight. But when allergy season was gone, I could relax and my perfect diet went out the window.

This happens to a lot of people. Some unhealthy condition motivates them to follow a healthful diet, and when they feel better or lose the extra weight, they relax and go back on a more delicious but less healthful diet.

To do anything perfectly is too much of a burden for anyone to carry!

While visiting the clinic for five days, I took the allergy treatment, and it worked dramatically. While I was there, I studied the other new treatments Dr. Hitt was researching. Taking advantage of his fifty years of research, I learned about the use of ozone therapy to cleanse the body of viruses and intravenous amino acid supplementation to normalize brain chemistry.

Every day in Dr. Hitt's clinic, I witnessed patients who stopped addictions without any withdrawal symptoms by means of intravenous amino acid supplementation. Patients could come in high on heroin or cocaine and leave in nine days free from addictive cravings.

During my allergy treatment, I met several of these patients. Many had begun to feel normal happiness for the first time in their lives. Tears of joy would come to their eyes as they shared how happy they were. For the first time in their lives, such patients were producing healthy amounts of brain chemicals. All their unhealthy cravings seemingly vanished. I do not know whether all the patients stayed off drugs, but in the short term the treatment seemed successful.

What I saw appeared miraculous. Although I had no addictions, I wondered what it might do for me.

For the first time in their lives, formerly addicted patients were producing healthy brain chemicals.

Dr. Hitt explained the basic ideas of ozone therapy and amino acid supplementation. Although I was healthy, my viral load was much higher than it had been when I was younger. We all start out with viruses in the body, but the immune system protects us from them. As we get older, the viruses gradually grow stronger and the immune system gets weaker. Ozone therapy provides more oxygen to the bloodstream, and this extra O_3 kills millions of harmful viruses, helping to strengthen the immune system. Thus the aging process is postponed. In the past, many movie stars would go to Mexico or Germany to get this expensive treatment to preserve their youthful looks and vitality. Now, with technological advances, the treatment is not expensive at all.

Dr. Hitt also pointed out that although most people don't suffer from such extreme symptoms of mental illness as depression or addiction, they might suffer from the same symptoms to a lesser degree. Through amino acid supplementation, they could increase the production of healthy brain chemicals and immediately begin to experience benefits as well.

As a personal experiment, I decided to try both treatments. I had no idea how profoundly I would be affected. After a couple of days of low energy associated with the elimination of toxins, I began to feel really good.

When I got home, I was very pleased. My allergies were gone, and I felt great. Mission accomplished. Although I had more energy and felt really good, I didn't feel *that* different. I was still me. I point this out because my wife couldn't believe what had happened. She said I was a different man . . . the man she fell in love with twenty-three years ago.

Without trying, I automatically became a better and more attentive husband. This change was so natural that I didn't even notice it. In my mind, I was already doing all the right things in my relationship. I love my wife, and we have a wonderful relationship. Since my work is about relationships, I knew what was required, and for the most part, I was very successful at it.

> Without trying, I automatically became
> a better and more attentive husband.

A few weeks after I returned home, my wife pointed out the changes. She noticed that I had started being more affectionate most of the time. I was more attentive to her. I was watching less TV. I was cleaning up after myself. I was helping out with the dishes all the time. I was remembering to take out the trash. I started making the bed. I cleaned out my closet. I washed my car. I was offering to help with things more of the time. I had more patience and didn't get frustrated as easily. I seemed genuinely interested in what she had to say. After her observations, I realized I had changed.

Wow, all that, and I didn't even try. I didn't even know I was doing it. From my perspective, I had always done all that good stuff. The big difference was frequency. Now I was doing it *all* the time.

SELECTIVE MEMORY

We men tend to have selective memory. We remember all the good things we do but have no recollection of the times when we forget and don't do those things. This was certainly true in my case. I thought I was *always* doing those things. Certainly I did them some of the time, particularly if my wife asked for my support. But now, after my return home, I was automatically doing the good things much of the time, and she wasn't even having to ask or remind me.

What I had noticed when I returned home was that my wife was much happier. I was not aware that I was doing so much more. What had happened?

What happened, as I learned from Dr. Hitt, was that my brain had started producing healthy brain chemicals. By feeding my brain the amino acids that it needed, I was automatically doing the things that I had done in the past as a result of *willpower* or as a response to my wife's request.

By accident, I had stumbled on a secret that not only made me feel good but also motivated me to give and receive more love and support in my relationship.

INSIGHT AND ENERGY

I had known what to do in a relationship, but now I had an abundance of energy to put those insights into practice. When your energy levels are low, even when you have the right insight, it takes a lot of effort to put into practice what you have learned. With lower levels of energy, you have to stop from time to time and rest. With the Mars-Venus relationship information and endless energy to put that insight into action, I found it easy to put into practice everything I had learned about love, communication, and relationships. My life changed completely.

When energy levels are low, sustaining the
romance in a relationship is hard work.

So many things came into focus. So many new answers flooded into my mind. Women have always asked why men have so much interest and passion in the beginning of the relationship, but then later, that passion diminishes. Though there are many valid answers to this question, ultimately it all comes down to brain chemistry.

For passion to be sustained, a relationship needs to be growing and changing. We are always more excited about a song when we first hear it. After we hear the recording over and over, it becomes less interesting. Seeing any movie five times, even one you love, can lead to boredom. This certainly explains why passion disappears in a relationship. Or does it?

The truth is that people are not recordings or movies; they are changing and growing much of the time. For most people, however, ordinary change over time is not enough stimulation to keep the passion alive. The routine of domestic life results in a kind of boredom or low-energy state in the relationship. What I discovered is that when brain chemistry is stimulated, the boredom goes away, and the energy or passion you felt in the beginning is restored. All that spontaneous passion we felt in the beginning returns, not because our partner is new and different, but because our brain chemistry has changed.

SUSTAINING HEALTHY BRAIN CHEMISTRY

About a month later, the effects of the treatment lessened. I started taking naps again. My wife noticed that the effects of the ozone therapy and the amino acid supplementation were wearing off. She suggested we look at my calendar and schedule another trip to Mexico. In the meantime, I started to research food supplements to stimulate my brain chemistry.

I began experimenting with a variety of health products that provided the essential amino acids that Dr. Hitt's treatment supplied. I also looked for the simplest program for cleansing the body and blood. I didn't want to depend on getting treatments in a hospital every few months.

What surfaced in my research were products specially designed to help children with attention deficit disorder (ADD) and attention deficit/hyperactivity disorder (ADHD). This made sense, because abundant research demonstrates that various kinds of amino acid supplementation help children with ADD and ADHD. The symptoms of these disorders were disappearing for both children and adults. Such products were an alternative to such prescription drugs as Ritalin.

Amino acid supplementation is helping both children and adults to stop taking Ritalin for ADD and ADHD symptoms.

During my search to find a natural way of getting amino acids to my brain and cleansing the body without needing a one-week intravenous treatment and ozone therapy, I eventually discovered a nutritional product that had many of the same effects for me. It was a nutrient-dense breakfast meal replacement powder that you blend with water. After my first drink, I could feel my brain starting to wake up again.

This meal replacement, rich in amino acids, was having the same effect on me as visiting Dr. Hitt's clinic in Mexico. Someone with a serious problem or a drug condition would probably need the medical intervention, but this breakfast shake provided what I needed. As I shared it with all my patients and friends, it worked for them as well to different degrees.

Some needed a little more time before they felt the effects. After all, I had already undergone the treatment in Mexico. Even that treatment takes several days. The difference between Dr. Hitt's treatment and a breakfast shake is the delivery system. When we drink amino acids, they are digested in the stomach and then processed by the liver. If the digestion is weak or the liver is toxic, then the amino acids are not fully converted into brain chemicals. Intravenous amino acid supplementation, however, bypasses a weak stomach or a toxic liver.

Intravenous amino acid supplementation bypasses a weak stomach or a toxic liver.

If one doesn't get the full benefit of oral amino acid supplementation, it is generally because the amino acids are not getting to the brain. That is why finding an effective cleansing program for the body and liver was another of my goals. Not everyone can go to Mexico to get ozone therapy to help the body get rid of toxins. The brand I used also included an effective process for cleansing the liver so it could more effectively process and convert the amino acids into the needed neurotransmitters.

Weak digestion or a toxic liver blocks the production of brain chemicals. Dr. Hitt's intravenous treatment works so dramatically because it is not dependent on the stomach to digest the proteins or the liver to process the amino acids. Through intravenous treatment, the stomach and liver are bypassed and the amino acids have direct access to the brain for the production of neural transmitters. If you strengthen your digestion with enzyme supplements and drink minerals and aloe vera to cleanse the liver, your body can more effectively digest proteins and fats so that the liver can process and convert amino acids into healthy brain chemistry.

WEIGHT LOSS OR RELATIONSHIP ENRICHMENT?

The amino acid shake and cleansing program I used is called Isagenix. It is advertised and promoted as an accelerated weight management program (www.roadtohealth.Isagenix.com or customer service at 1-877-877-8111). Although I was looking for a natural food supplement to produce healthy brain chemistry and not weight loss, I tried their product. To my delight, it worked. In a few days, the many benefits of amino acid supplementation were back. As a side effect, I also lost weight.

I started their accelerated weight loss program and lost nine pounds in nine days. A few weeks later, I lost another six pounds and arrived back at my ideal weight. Although weight loss was not the reason I started this program, it was a great side effect. Now I had more energy for my relationship *and* I looked great.

It was easy to lose weight, because the amino acid supplementation took away all cravings for extra food. Correct brain chemistry gives us relaxation and endless energy. With this support for our brain, we stop overeating to get more energy or to find comfort. Just as amino acid supplementation can free drug addicts from their drug cravings, it can free anyone from hunger cravings for unhealthy food during the day. It is so liberating to feel no urge to overeat and no cravings during the day for junk food snacks.

JUNK FOOD AND ADDICTION

Junk food cravings are just another form of addiction. They give us quick energy and comfort, but the results are temporary. Very quickly, the production of brain chemicals lessens, and then we hunger for more junk food. When the production of brain hormones drops shortly after a meal of nutrient-deficient food, we crave more junk food again. When our brain chemistry is off, one cookie is never enough.

When our brain chemistry is off,
one cookie is never enough.

Aside from accelerated weight loss, the thousands of people who have tried the Isagenix program have reported freedom from hunger cravings, as well as stable moods, more energy, and better sleep. These are all characteristic of a balanced brain. At this point in my journey, I stopped testing other products and focused on finding out what made this product work so well.

REVERSE ENGINEERING

In the world of inventions and innovations, the secret to success is reverse engineering. Find a product that works, take it apart to find out why it works, then see if you can improve on it. By examining all the ingredients, I realized that with the proper insight, any person could go to his or her health food store to gather the ingredients needed. In addition, I felt if this product could be integrated into a program that included the unique needs of men and women, it could be even more effective.

With the proper insight, any person could simply go to his or her health food store to gather the ingredients needed.

In Chapter 9, I will provide you with a list of these supplements, which are available at most health food stores or nutrition centers. By combining these ingredients into your morning breakfast routine, you will begin to get results right away. If at any time while reading this book you are ready to begin the program, I recommend going to Chapter 9 and starting right away. You can always come back and read Chapters 2 to 8.

To find out why this product was so effective, I went right to the source. I flew to Phoenix to meet John Anderson, the man who developed Isagenix. In the past twenty-three years, he has manufactured more than a billion dollars' worth of health products for over 250 brands. Frustrated by the reported low quality in many health supplements, he came out of retirement to provide the highest quality health products he could manufacture. Combining into one program the various healthy elements that have worked dramatically in different brands, he developed Isagenix health products.

John Anderson has manufactured health products not just for hundreds of public brands, but privately as well for famous athletes, boxers, and many major football teams. The best coaches know that nutritional supplementation is essential for peak performance.

The best coaches know that nutritional supplementation is essential for peak performance.

By taking the ingredients of different successful programs and combining them into one, he developed the Isagenix accelerated weight management program.

John Anderson openly shared all his secrets with me. He showed me all the different ingredients. He explained that he had manufactured products for a variety of lines that were successful for some people but not for all. The success of any program increases when it meets your specific needs. If I am deficient in vitamins and you are not, then a program to supplement those vitamins would be more effective for me and less effective for you. Similarly, different programs would work well for some people, but not as well for others whose needs were different. Each program would have its own emphasis. Here is a brief summary of his program:

1. Amino acid supplementation to increase energy, stabilize mood, and improve mental capacity
2. A full range of vitamin supplements and/or herbs to help the body cleanse and heal itself
3. Enzyme supplements and trace minerals to strengthen digestion and increase vitality
4. A breakfast meal replacement blended shake, with a particular balance of protein, fat, and carbohydrate to provide healthy weight management and peak performance

Although John Anderson's focus was to provide a healthy weight management solution, he has also developed a general program for good health, which includes producing healthy brain chemistry.

To create the brain chemistry of health, happiness, and lasting romance, I personally use and recommend using the Isagenix products as a part of the Mars and Venus Solution. You can, however, achieve similar results by going to your health food store and selecting the different ingredients and putting them together yourself. Even if you choose to use the Isagenix brand for the nutritional part of this program, you will still need to make a trip to the health food store to get some additional ingredients.

LIVING IN THE ZONE

Once you begin *The Mars and Venus Diet and Exercise Solution*, your brain will start producing a balance of feel-good chemicals. After this change is complete, you will have the ability to listen correctly to your body. To know what foods put your brain out of balance, you first have to experience what it feels like to be in balance. When you are, you will know what foods throw you out of balance.

With *The Mars and Venus Diet and Exercise Solution*, you will experience a mind/body state of consistent energy and well-being. This state is what Barry Sears popularized in his diet book *Enter the Zone*. He described the zone as a peak performance state in which everything seems to go your way, a state in which he claims "your body and mind work together at their ultimate best." By eating the right nutrients for breakfast, you will very quickly begin to live in this zone.

When your brain chemicals are balanced, you enter a zone of consistent energy and well-being.

In my twenties, I would enter this state by practicing yoga and meditation. But after eating a meal, I would quickly fall out. I didn't realize it was the meal that took me out of the zone. I thought I just needed more meditation practice to sustain this positive state. I spent years trying to perfect this state so that it would last all the time. Little did I know then that if I had supplemented my diet with amino acids and other nutrients, I could have sustained that state. Certainly all that yoga had other benefits, but it could have been a lot easier and much more fun.

Then I spent my thirties learning to create love and lasting romance in my marriage. When the romantic hormones were being stimulated, I was in the zone, but when there were communication problems, I was out of the zone once again. Little did I know that it was my diet that kept me from sustaining the romantic and loving feelings I had in my heart.

In my forties, I would enter this state through my work. All I had to do was speak on TV or radio or stand in front of an audience, and I would go into a heightened state. During that time, I wrote twelve books. Each time I sat down to write a book, I would go into the zone and write at exceptionally high speeds. Certainly, developing ideas for a book takes years, but once those ideas were in place, the actual writing only took a couple of months. I was at the peak of creative energy.

Yet after a stimulating seminar, a media appearance, or a day of writing, within a short period of time, my energy and mood would drop. When faced with the challenge of work, like all men with low dopamine levels, I would rev up and my energy would rise. Since my diet was not balanced and fortified with essential nutrients, I would crash and become exhausted.

Now I am in my fifties, and I live with balanced brain chemistry all the time, and what a difference it makes. With a balanced diet, I don't crash after stimulating work projects or intimate time with my wife. The good feelings from prayer, meditation, and exercise are consistent. Certainly I still do regular practices to keep my mind, body, and spirit attuned to an elevated state, but without a balanced diet and exercise program, I would still lose that highly charged feeling.

Good diet and exercise make good feelings consistent.

I live in a peak state all the time—until I don't. Occasionally I will eat the wrong foods or forget to eat and then lose it. Fortunately, three hours later, by correcting my food balance, I am easily back in form, with plenty of energy for work, my wife, my children, and my life.

Extreme stress and not enough sleep also can disrupt that state. I usually have so much energy that it is easy to go without sleep, but that takes a toll. It is very important, particularly in the beginning of this program, that you go to bed early and rise early.

Research has shown that the brain produces serotonin most efficiently for the two hours after sunrise. This is particularly important for women, who commonly have low serotonin levels. For men, getting to bed early is most important. It is during the two hours before midnight that the brain produces ample supplies of dopamine for the next day.

The brain continues to be productive, but these times are the most important and need to be observed whenever possible. I certainly don't limit myself to this routine, but it is my ideal schedule. With a good backup supply of dopamine in your sleep bank, you can afford to stay up late sometimes.

Most of the habits we cherish are based on limited brainpower. As your brain chemistry becomes balanced, give yourself permission to try new schedules as well as new eating routines. If programs have not worked for you in the past, they didn't balance your brain chemistry. It was not a symptom of weak will. Your program was not the solution for you.

Fortunately, it is never too late to learn to apply something new and good in your life. The great news is that we are designed to live in the zone. With the strong foundation of a healthy body, we can easily sustain the ideal mental and emotional states we have nurtured throughout our lives.

At any age, by eating the right balance of nutrients every morning, you will start the day by ensuring that the results you have been working so hard to achieve will stabilize and be consistent. The spirit inspires, the mind directs, the heart responds, but the body sustains us. It is our foundation. It provides the solid base for all the positive changes we wish to make in our mind, heart, and spirit.

As you begin to feel vibrant and energetic all the time, the particular foods, quantities, and combinations best for you become apparent. You will not depend on books and diet plans, but on your brain and body. How will you know? You will know by how you feel!

When a meal puts your body in balance, your energy stays high until your next meal. Some of the most common symptoms of this balanced state are endless energy, unconditional happiness, and unlimited love. If you live in this state, it is not only easier to pick and choose the right foods, but your relationships are easier as well.

ENDLESS ENERGY

Endless energy means having plenty of energy all the time, without naps, and feeling motivated to do things all the time. It is easy to get up in the morning, and you want to exercise. For men, when your wife asks you to empty the trash or to get up and do something, it is not a problem. When she talks more than you would prefer, instead of resisting, you feel, "I can do this."

With endless energy, you are able to listen, which manifests as patience and interest. When a man has lower levels of energy, he tries to rush a woman to the point and get to the solution. Focusing on a solution gives men energy. If a man has plenty of energy, he is not in such a hurry to get to the point or solve the problem.

When a woman feels tired and overwhelmed because she has too much to do, she has fallen from the zone of endless energy. In the zone, you don't sink into feelings of exhaustion, but instead can easily relax and ask for help. When a woman suffers from low energy, she often feels hopeless and depressed. Even if she does think about reaching out and asking for a little support, in her mind this thought is immediately countered by the thought, "It is more trouble than it is worth." As a result, she continues taking on more than she can do until she is exhausted.

Just the thought of how much she has to do makes her tired. This resistance to asking for help is another symptom of low energy.

UNCONDITIONAL HAPPINESS

Unconditional happiness means you smile for no reason at all, except for being alive. Certainly, life has its ups and downs, but through it all you are happy. This happiness is not an abstract concept but a tangible feeling that pervades your life with such emotions as enthusiasm, excitement, joy, and pleasure. Put simply: Even little things make you happy, and big problems don't knock you over. At difficult and challenging times, when things upset you, you are quickly able to come back to a warm feeling of gratitude for the good things in your life. In the bigger context of all the good in your life, the negative no longer has a grip on your mood.

Unconditional happiness means little things make you happy and big problems don't knock you over.

Unconditional happiness doesn't mean that you are not dependent on circumstance to make you happy. Whatever the circumstances, good or bad, you are rooted in your ability to see the whole picture. You don't drop into a depressed state by focusing on the negative and forgetting all the good in your life. Whenever someone is unhappy or depressed, that person has temporarily forgotten the good things about his or her situation.

In the zone of unconditional happiness, you may feel sad or disappointed after a loss, but not unhappy. You may feel angry and frustrated when you don't like what has happened, but not unloving. You may feel afraid in the face of loss or danger, but you are still in touch with your inner confidence. To be courageous does not mean you have no fear. It means you act in spite of your fears.

All imbalanced mental states—worry, hate, anxiety, depression, for example—result from focusing on the negative in life to the exclusion of the positive. These states of imbalance can now be measured by brain SPECT imaging, which gives a picture of the imbalance of activity in the brain. Different parts of your brain become overactive or underactive. With balanced brain chemistry you are able to see the whole picture and avoid focusing on the negative.

No matter how bad things get, there are still many things to be grateful for. If you are in balance and things upset you, you quickly regain your balance by feeling the positive feelings as well.

No matter how bad things get, there are still many things to be grateful for.

Experiencing unconditional happiness is like lying in a warm bathtub and enjoying the waves of pleasure that come from moving in the water or feeling the water move over you. Some things make you more or less happy, but you are always connected to your essential nature, which is to be happy. When the water is still, you may even forget that it is warm, but once there is movement you feel it again. Likewise, you may forget you are happy, but all it takes is doing something enjoyable and a wave of happiness fills your being with joy and gratitude.

UNLIMITED LOVE

Unlimited love doesn't mean that you love everyone equally. It means that you have so much love that you are not stingy with it. If someone disappoints you, you have so much love in your heart that you don't close your heart or withhold your love. Many times in relationships, we love each other when our partner is giving us what we want, but if she stops, we stop loving. The real test of love is whether you can continue to feel loving kindness for your partner even when he is not in a good mood or she is blaming you.

> The real test of love is whether you can
> continue to feel loving kindness even when
> you have been rejected!

As you begin to live with unlimited love, you will find that even when differences between people show up, creating tension and conflict, you are able to find the patience, kindness, and understanding to resolve misunderstanding and sustain the loving connection you choose to have with someone. You see the good in things and you stay motivated to share yourself.

Even in business, this is important. I do what I love to do, and if others don't always appreciate me, I am able to come back to sharing myself again, doing what I love to do.

When you withhold your love, you are the one who suffers the most. Ultimately, our most painful moments in life have to do with holding back the love in our hearts we are born to share. By learning to balance your brain chemistry and live in the zone of unlimited love, you will not only be healthy and happy, but you will experience a lifetime of love.

EVEN LOVE CAN HURT

When we love someone, we are actually much more vulnerable to being hurt. When we don't care about someone, they can't hurt us. The more we care, the easier it is for our feelings to be hurt. So many times couples truly love each other, but they get hurt as a result of misunderstanding.

> The closer we are, the easier it is to get hurt.

Feeling hurt occurs when we feel an imbalance of giving and receiving. We give our hearts, and our partner doesn't give back. We do something special, and our partner doesn't seem to care, and we feel taken for granted and unappreciated. We care for their needs, but they don't seem to care for ours. We love them, but they don't seem to love us as much. This imbalance causes hurt.

The real cause of this hurt is that when we determine that we are not getting what we deserve, we either stop giving our love to the person or to ourselves. When we are rejected by someone we love, we may conclude that we are inadequate or unworthy. This limiting belief is painful and causes us to feel hurt. Or we react to rejection by rejecting back. In one moment, we were loving ourselves and our partner, and in the next, we are rejected and we choose to reject back. We hold back our love, and as a result, we are the ones who suffer.

Pain arises when we close our hearts to others and to ourselves.

We are always happiest when we are loving others and loving ourselves: Feeling good about others and ourselves is a symptom of an open heart with unlimited love.

IT ALWAYS STARTS OUT AS SMALL STUFF

When we think about relationship problems, we often think about the big problems. The truth is, the little problems are most important. All big problems start out as small ones. When little misunderstandings are avoided or at least corrected, the big problems don't usually occur. If they do occur, by handling the little problems first, the big ones are then more easily solved. The secret for creating lasting love and romance is in resolving all the little problems, which are usually just misunderstandings.

The secret for creating lasting love and romance is in resolving the little problems.

With each misunderstanding, whether we know it or not, we get our feelings hurt. With a little time, our hurt feelings will heal like a physical bruise does. If we keep poking at the bruise, it will never heal. Instead, it will get worse. In a relationship, we will inevitably get bruised or bruise our partners. Everyone makes mistakes. Even the best dancer occasionally steps on a partner's foot.

To facilitate healing, we can learn to accept imperfection by practicing forgiveness, but we must also learn from our mistakes. Ultimately, when a man doesn't have the information to learn from his mistakes, he thinks something is wrong with his partner for feeling hurt, and he stops caring about correcting his mistakes. Likewise, when a woman doesn't understand men, she will close down, doubting that she can ever get what she needs in her relationship.

When differences show up, we mistakenly think something is wrong with our partners.

When a man comes home and his wife doesn't seem to appreciate him, he stops caring as much about doing the little things as he did in the beginning of the relationship. When he stops caring to do the little things, she stops appreciating him the way she did in the beginning. This lack of warm feelings causes an increasing tension that intensifies when they are trying to resolve normal differences or solve the normal problems that occur when two people share responsibilities.

Most of this tension starts with very simple misunderstandings. These misunderstandings arise because we speak different languages: men speak Martian and women speak Venusian. Here is an example:

Both come home from work and she says, "Do you want to go out?"

He says, "No, let's stay home. We can just eat leftovers."

She thinks, "He is so selfish. All he thinks about is himself. He doesn't care for me the way he used to. If he did, he'd want to go out."

As a result of this simple interaction, they eat leftovers and she begins to pull back and close her heart. As a direct result, she will become a bit indifferent to him. When he attempts to get close that night, she may not be in the mood, and as a result of this rejection, his heart closes a little as well. Life goes on, but their positive feelings of love and connection are a little less strong.

Little hurts block the growth of love and connection.

In this little mishap, she is annoyed with him, because he didn't offer to take her out to dinner. In her language, by saying, "Do you want to go out?" she was saying, "I am in the mood for going out to dinner. Let's go out."

This is what she meant, but what he heard her saying is, "I don't really care what we do tonight. Would you like to go out or stay home or what? I will be happy to do whatever you want."

When I explain this to men, they generally respond by saying something like, "If that is what she meant, then why didn't she just say it?"

Well, that is exactly what she did say but in Venusian. Any woman would have correctly interpreted her meaning.

ROMANCE AND BRAIN CHEMISTRY

Most men get a taste of balanced brain chemistry whenever they are turned on and expecting to be romantically intimate. For a man, being in the mood for romance activates balanced brain chemistry. If his diet and exercise program do not sustain this state, he falls out of his high and goes to sleep after his needs are met. This is not his fault, nor is it a sign that he doesn't care for her. It is simply that his diet cannot support sustained passion and energy.

For a man, being in the mood for romance
activates a taste for peak experience.

When a woman is happily being romanced, she will begin to experience balanced brain chemistry as well. This is why women's magazines are so focused on how to create romance, or more important, on how to look, communicate, or dress in a way that inspires and stimulates a man's romantic interest in her. A man's romantic desire to please her, at least in the beginning of a relationship, can and does give her unlimited happiness. When he falls out of that state, she does, too. This kind of dependency is not healthy for a relationship.

With a balanced diet and exercise program that keeps her in a peak state, a woman is not so vulnerable to the moods of her partner. She is able to appreciate and enjoy when he demonstrates his romantic affections, but she doesn't feel needy or unhappy when he is in his cave. She has plenty of other activities to stimulate her positive feelings. Instead of needing him to feel good and loving, she already feels that way. As her dependence on him for fulfillment diminishes, the potential for tension lessens and communication of needs becomes much easier.

With unlimited happiness and unconditional love,
a woman is not so dependent on her partner to
feel happy and in love.

Women, when you want something from a man and there is no emotional change, neediness, or tone of demand associated with your request, he is much more inclined to say yes.

Men, when you interact with your partner with greater energy, attention, and warmth, you will get the loving responses you enjoyed in the beginning of your relationship. By having the natural energy and enthusiasm you had in the past, you will bring back the old feeling in your relationship.

For both Mars and Venus, as your diet and exercise program

help you sustain a high level of energy and well-being, making a relationship work stops being work.

WHERE SHOULD WE EAT?

While we are on the topic of food, let's look at a simple example of how Mars and Venus misunderstand each other. In this scenario, he comes home and she is more direct and says, "Let's go out to dinner tonight."

He responds by saying, "Okay, where would you like to go?"

In a friendly tone, she says, "Umm, I don't know."

Happy to take charge and solve the problem, he says, "Okay, let's go to D'angelo's for Italian food."

She takes a moment to reflect and then says, "I don't know, I'm not in the mood for Italian. We had pasta yesterday."

He says, "Okay, let's go to Jennie Low's for Chinese food. We always enjoy eating there."

Happy to have a conversation about restaurants and food, she says pleasantly, "No, I want something different tonight."

He says with a tone of slight frustration, "Okay, let's get burritos at Lucinda's."

Once again, she innocently expresses her next feeling and says, "No, we had Mexican food on Monday."

To which he responds with annoyance, "Okay, I don't care. You decide. Let's just go!"

For the rest of the evening, there is tension between them. She feels he doesn't care about her, and he feels no matter what he does, it is not enough to make her happy. He doesn't feel appreciated and begins to withhold his warm and friendly feelings. She feels he was too impatient, abrupt, and uncaring. As a result, she pulls away and becomes a little cold and distant. Both of them have closed their hearts.

As this dynamic continues for months and years, they eventually may open their hearts to strangers, but their hearts are closed to each other. They may love each other, but they no longer feel that love. Instead, they begin to take each other for granted and gradually grow apart. Some couples just become comfortable. They learn to accept each other by lowering their expectations, but the passion and romance are gone.

Sometimes couples learn to accept each other by lowering their expectations.

With the insight of Mars and Venus, a man realizes that it can be fun and relaxing for a woman just to talk about where they could eat. If my wife and daughters want to discuss in great detail all the options before making a decision, I now realize that this is a little Venusian ritual they perform to relax and feel good. In scientific terms, as they share and explore the problem together and then collaborate to come up with a solution, their feel-good hormones and brain chemicals are being produced. By effectively solving the problem and succeeding in supporting the woman he loves, a man can also experience feel-good hormones in his body and brain.

In this case, instead of becoming frustrated, an aware, balanced man versed in Mars and Venus insights will have the patience and the wisdom to participate in the process. What follows is an example of participating to stimulate positive hormones in her brain and body.

She says, "Where should we go?"

He suggests the Italian restaurant. She then responds, "I don't know, I'm not in the mood for Italian. We had pasta yesterday."

He then comments, "Yeah, I really like their angel hair spaghetti, but every day is too much. Let's go to Jennie Low's for Chinese food. We always enjoy eating there."

Happy to have a conversation about restaurants, she says, "No, I want something different tonight. I don't think I want tofu tonight. I need something else. I wonder what?"

He says in a friendly tone, sensing that he is making her happy by having this conversation, "Well, we certainly don't have to have Chinese. We might want to have Chinese food when we go out to lunch with the Browns next Wednesday. Maybe we should just get takeout from Lucinda's?"

With warmth and appreciation for having such a cooperative and supportive husband, she replies, "I don't think I want a tostado tonight. And besides that, I would rather let someone else do the dishes and have a sit-down dinner. I don't want to get takeout."

Having patiently waited to make a decisive statement, he then makes his masterful close. By taking some time to consider her feelings, he then can take charge and pick a restaurant. He then says, "Okay, I've got a good idea, let's go to the other Mexican restaurant and eat there. You can get your favorite fish tacos."

At this point, she is melting in his warmth and consideration. She feels so supported by and supportive to him. Not only is he taking time, but he is engaged in the three things that help stimulate balanced brain chemistry in women. He is communicating, cooperating, and collaborating. She then responds, "Okay, great idea, let's do it."

He is also feeling great. By applying his insight with effective communication skills, he is generating the ideal brain chemistry for a man. Men need to sense they are getting something done to feel good. A sense of action, achievement, and accomplishment puts him in the mood for romance as well. When they get home, her response to his romantic gestures will be the same: "Okay, great idea, let's do it!"

KNOWLEDGE, DIET, AND EXERCISE

These misunderstandings that I have explored in all my Mars and Venus books occur all the time between men and women. They are little, but feelings of resistance and resentment may accumulate over time. Even with a good diet and exercise, these misunderstandings can lessen the love and passion in a relationship. It is essential that we have not only a diet that sustains the

love in our hearts but also the knowledge to make our relationships work.

I don't want to imply that diet alone can make your relationships work. Knowledge is essential. Without a better understanding of our differences and good communication skills, little
problems, which could be easily solved, eventually turn into bigger problems that we think can't be solved—big problems such
as:

"I just don't have feelings for you anymore."

"I am not turned on to you anymore."

"I give and I give and I have nothing left to give."

"No matter what I do, it is never enough! I give up."

Even these big problems can often be resolved with some
Mars and Venus relationship coaching or counseling, and a good
diet and exercise program. As a counselor for thirty years, I have
consistently helped couples and individuals to resolve big relationship issues. With these same Mars and Venus skills, hundreds of coaches and counselors help thousands of people every
day to resolve such problems.

With the passage of time, some problems come back. A par-
tial relapse is not from a lack of knowledge but from a lack of
energy, happiness, and love in the heart. Often, a relapse has
less to do with a lack of knowledge and more to do with diet
and exercise. If you are depressed, you may love your partner,
but you cannot feel it or be stimulated by it.

**If you are depressed, you may love your partner
but you cannot feel it or be stimulated by it.**

Without knowledge and a healthy diet and exercise routine,
you will find it difficult to create lasting love, passion, and romance. I know, because at times it has taken tremendous willpower for me to overcome challenges in my own relationship. I
have worked hard at making my marriage work, and it has been
worth it.

A common cliché of relationship advice is "Keeping the romance alive takes hard work." This was certainly true for me. I have great respect for those who have been willing to put in the hard work. If it takes hard work for someone who is a relationship expert to create lasting romance, think how much harder it is for those who have other jobs and expertise.

In retrospect, it would have been much easier if my diet and exercise routine for all those years had been more supportive. When your diet and exercise program supplies you with a positive outlook and great energy, the work of building and susataining a relationship becomes much easier.

When you experience unlimited love, it is so much easier to apologize for your mistakes and forgive your partner for his or hers. You have the energy to give more to your partner even on those days when he or she has less to give to you. When you are happier, you are able to let go of misunderstandings and mishaps, rather than hold on to them. With endless energy, unconditional happiness, and unlimited love, you can easily put into practice the things you have learned that make a relationship work.

By integrating the ideas and insights of *Men Are from Mars, Women Are from Venus* with the most up-to-date programs and innovations in health today, you will have the keys to live a long and happy life. By learning the simple steps to changing your brain chemistry, you will awaken your potential to make your dreams come true.

3

DOPAMINE IS FROM MARS

Dopamine is a chemical in the brain that gives us energy and motivation. Serotonin is another brain chemical that relaxes us and helps us to remember everything is going to be all right. These important brain chemicals are produced from specific amino acids contained in the proteins we eat. By directly changing brain chemistry with *The Mars and Venus Diet and Exercise Solution,* men and women can relax and enjoy their relationships more.

By increasing serotonin production in women and dopamine production in men, we are much more capable of applying all the good communication skills we have learned to support the people we love most. Men and women process the amino acids they eat in their proteins very differently. The end result of a nutritionally deficient diet is that men often have a dopamine deficiency and women a serotonin deficiency. Dopamine is from Mars because most men tend to be deficient in it. When you are deficient in dopamine, then naturally you seek out behaviors that stimulate the production of more dopamine. For example, men are drawn to sports, action movies, and dangerous activities because they stimulate dopamine. The lower a man's levels of dopamine, the more he depends on these activities to feel energized. The comfort and security of relationships stimulates serotonin.

Men don't think of relationships as much as women do because men generally have plenty of serotonin.

Research reveals that the male brain actually synthesizes serotonin 52 percent faster than the female brain and can store twice as much as well. By eating a diet designed to produce dopamine, a man will have the potential for much more energy and motivation.

Men's brains actually synthesize serotonin 52 percent faster than women's brains and can store twice as much as well.

Serotonin is from Venus because most women are deficient in it. Low levels of serotonin create a health crisis for women, just as low levels of dopamine create a health crisis for men. Low levels of serotonin are associated with overgiving in relationships, food cravings, and depression. Serotonin is primarily produced in the morning. By adding a healthy exercise and breakfast routine, women can produce plenty of serotonin every day.

For both men and women, however, a healthy diet and exercise program on its own is not enough to create the brain chemistry of health, happiness, and lasting romance. A complete nutritional and exercise program only provides the *potential* for creating healthy brain chemistry. But it takes better communication in our relationships to stimulate that potential. One program without the other is ineffective; they are completely interdependent.

NEUROTRANSMITTERS AND BRAIN DAMAGE

Neurotransmitters are hormones in the brain required for communication between brain cells. In order to function as it is designed to, the brain, just like a car, needs gas and water in the radiator. Without ample production of neurotransmitters, the brain becomes overactive in some places and underactive in others. Without the gas (dopamine), it is underactive in areas; without water in the radiator (serotonin), it becomes overheated or overactive in areas.

Brain researchers have long known that symptoms of mental illness are the direct result of brain imbalances. This insight can now be directly verified with modern technology. The activity of the brain can be photographed and even observed in real time. Symptoms of depression, anxiety, anger, addiction, and overwhelm can be directly linked to an imbalance of activity in different parts of the brain. This is brilliantly explored by Daniel G. Amen, M.D., in his book *Change Your Brain, Change Your Life.*

This imbalance is sometimes caused by actual brain damage from an accident, traumatic stress, or some genetic defect. In these cases, the use of prescribed psychoactive medications sometimes helps to restore healthy brain balance by stimulating the production of serotonin or dopamine in the brain. With the production of missing neurotransmitters, the brain comes back into balance and symptoms may disappear. There are many important neurotransmitters in the brain, but for our purposes we will focus on the two most important ones: serotonin and dopamine. Some brain researchers also believe that these two key brain chemicals modulate the activity of all the other neurotransmitters. The functions of these neuromodulators are explored in great detail by Ronald A. Ruden, M.D., in his book *The Craving Brain.* Let's explore two common examples: a deficiency of dopamine or serotonin.

By stimulating the production of missing
neurotransmitters, the brain comes
back into balance.

The first example has to do with a deficiency of dopamine. The common symptoms of ADD or ADHD are all associated with an underactive prefrontal cortex and a deficiency of dopamine. The prefrontal cortex occupies the front third of the brain, underneath the forehead. It provides us with the capacity to make goals and plans and to carry them out. Children with low dopamine and an underactive prefrontal cortex tend to be easily bored and seek out stimulation from new and different sensations or experiences that create an immediate response. They can easily give attention to something that engages them.

When children have low levels of dopamine, mothers and teachers often complain that their children don't listen and tend to do what they want to do rather than consider the needs of others. When required to focus on something that doesn't seem relevant or to the point, their brains begin to shut down. They often seek immediate gratification, require extra stimulation, and lose interest very quickly. With increasing attempts to focus, these children deplete dopamine supplies and demonstrate symptoms ranging from boredom, tiredness, and restlessness to hyperactivity, impulsiveness, and disruptiveness.

By taking a dopamine-stimulating drug like Ritalin, children and adults can experience dramatically reduced symptoms. With more dopamine available, the brain begins to function normally and the prefrontal cortex becomes more active, even with brain damage. With increased dopamine, the patient experiences to different degrees a surge in clarity, pleasure, energy, and motivation. A brain fog lifts, and the sometimes indefinable flatness of boredom is forgotten as a person is suddenly much more interested in responding to the needs of others. With the help of dopamine, a person suddenly has a renewed sense of meaning and purpose.

With increased dopamine, the patient experiences a surge in clarity, pleasure, energy, and motivation.

The second example has to do with a deficiency of serotonin. Common symptoms of depression are most often associated with low serotonin and an overactive limbic system in the brain. The limbic system is located in the center of the brain. This part of the brain sets our emotional tone. When it becomes over-active, this is correlated with depression and negativity.

Increasing serotonin levels help to relax an overactive brain. By taking a serotonin-stimulating drug like Prozac, a person can dramatically reduce the symptoms of depression. Common symptoms of depression are moodiness, and feeling hopeless, helpless, worthless, pessimistic, guilty, or unable to let go of the past and be fully present.

Depression is often overlooked in young girls, because when the depression is mild, these symptoms tend to promote coop-erative or "good" behavior. A deficiency of serotonin often leads to an overresponsiveness to the needs of others. These children care too much about the needs of others and often have difficulty asking for what they want. It is common not only for women but also for their daughters to feel overwhelmed, as though there is too much to do and not enough time or support to do it. These symptoms will vary according to the temperament of the child.

With more serotonin, the limbic system relaxes, and the symptoms of depression are alleviated. With increased serotonin, the patient experiences a wave of calm, comfort, and fulfillment. The turbulent storm of automatic negative thoughts subsides; the sometimes indefinable feeling of abandonment is forgotten; and she is freed from the gripping experience of past hurts. With the help of serotonin, a person is able to let go of the past and live in the present, with a healthy optimism about the future.

With increased serotonin, the patient experiences a wave of calm, comfort, and fulfillment.

Without the right diet and exercise, a healthy brain is unable to synthesize adequate amounts of neurotransmitters, and as a result it begins to appear as if it was damaged.

As millions of children have now been diagnosed with ADD and ADHD, clearly brain damage or some genetic flaw is not at the root of the problem. These millions of children are experiencing the symptoms of the same problems that most adults are facing: the symptoms of dopamine and serotonin deficiency. This imbalance of brain chemistry is primarily caused by nutritional deficiency. When adjustments are made in diet and exercise, along with changes in lifestyle that promote the stimulation of dopamine and serotonin through better communication, normal brain functioning has been restored for thousands.

LOW LEVELS OF DOPAMINE

As we explore the symptoms of low dopamine syndrome, it will become increasingly clear that dopamine deficiency is from Mars. A woman can experience some of the symptoms of low dopamine, but they are not as common or dramatic. When a woman does exhibit symptoms of low levels of dopamine, the Mars and Venus Solution for her is the same as it is for women with low levels of serotonin. The problem is nutritional deficiency. The solution has nothing to do with her specific imbalance. This Mars and Venus Solution fuels and supports her body in restoring and healing itself to produce the correct balance of chemicals for her. It is not necessary for her or for you to figure out your brain imbalances.

We know low dopamine syndrome is from Mars, because children with ADD and ADHD all have low levels of dopamine, and 90 percent of these millions of children afflicted with ADD and ADHD are boys! Most criminals demonstrate extreme symptoms of low dopamine syndrome, and 90 percent of criminals in jail are men.

Ninety percent of the millions of children afflicted with ADD and ADHD are boys!

One out of every five boys is diagnosed with this disorder. Consider that for every boy diagnosed with this disorder, there are probably two more who are borderline. The two remaining boys probably demonstrate the same symptoms but with less consistency. This disorder is a national epidemic.

The same holds true for men. As a relationship counselor, I have been able to identify the common symptoms of boys with this disorder in almost all the men I have met or counseled. Take any common attribute in men that frustrates women, magnify it, and you have a list of the symptoms of low dopamine syndrome. With lower levels of dopamine, these symptoms are magnified.

Take any common attribute in men that frustrates women, magnify it, and you have the symptoms of low dopamine syndrome.

A syndrome is a collection of symptoms that are associated with a particular condition. Not all the symptoms need be present for one to experience low dopamine syndrome. A syndrome shows up in different ways for different people because people have such a range of temperaments.

A syndrome shows up in different ways for different people because people have such a range of temperaments.

This means that even though you may not exhibit all of the symptoms, you may still have low dopamine levels. Think of it this way: If you were carrying a substantial financial debt, your reaction could easily be different from another person's. One person might ask for help, another might take medications to sleep at night, another might change jobs, another might borrow money, another might get more education, another might work overtime, another might sell some property, another might cut back on expenses, another might seek counseling, take a seminar, or read a self-help book, and another might go on vacation to reevaluate his life. These reactions would then be the different symptoms of one condition—financial debt, or "high debt syndrome." One person might have many of the symptoms or just a few.

In addition, a symptom will be more or less consistent or intense depending on the degree of deficiency and your diet and exercise routine. It is not an all-or-nothing phenomenon. If you eat well one day but poorly the next, then your symptoms will be inconsistent and will vary.

WHAT STIMULATES DOPAMINE

Generally speaking, whenever a man has an opportunity to protect, serve, or make a difference, dopamine is stimulated in his brain. If he suffers from low dopamine syndrome, it means that normal opportunities to protect, serve, and make a difference are not enough to stimulate healthy dopamine levels and the energy and pleasure associated with those levels. To get enough energy and pleasure, he requires more or excess stimulation.

When a man's brain is not producing enough dopamine, he has to turn up the volume. Instead of getting in his car to go for a drive, he has to race his car. Instead of locking the doors in his home to protect his family, he needs to buy a gun and practice shooting it regularly. Instead of riding his bike for an hour or two, he needs to ride four hours a day. Instead of watching his favorite team on TV, he has to watch every team. Instead of being turned on by his wife, he spends hours checking out pornography on the Web. Instead of being satisfied making a good living, he has to make more and more money.

Ultimately, a man requires a certain amount of risk, challenge, and competition to stimulate dopamine. If he has healthy levels of dopamine production in his brain, the daily opportunities to protect, serve, and make a difference are enough to give him energy and pleasure. When his dopamine levels are low, emptying the trash just doesn't do it, but making a lot of money does. With this insight, a woman can begin to understand why a man will remember to make a business call but will forget to empty the trash.

Ultimately, a man requires a certain amount
of risk, challenge, and competition to
stimulate dopamine.

SYMPTOMS OF LOW DOPAMINE SYNDROME

Here are twelve common symptoms of the dopamine deficiency
syndrome compared with symptoms of healthy dopamine production:

1. Low Energy at Home

With low dopamine levels, a man has lots of energy and passion
at work, but when he comes home, he is tired and experiences
lower levels of energy and motivation. Yet if a call comes from
the office, he is suddenly animated and fully alive. The new and
different challenges of his work stimulate dopamine, but the
comfortable routine at home does not.

Work easily stimulates dopamine,
but marriage doesn't.

With normal dopamine levels, a man does not require the
stimulation of new and different challenges to give him energy.
When he comes home, he is easily stimulated by the challenges
of raising a family and helping out with domestic activities.

To nurture the production of dopamine in her husband, a
woman can be responsive to his actions, achievements, and ac-
complishments, no matter how small. Her trusting comments
and appreciative responses to his efforts, along with acceptance
for who he is, can most effectively stimulate dopamine.

If his dopamine levels are low, no amount of appreciation,
acceptance, or trust will be enough. A wife or loving partner can
stimulate the production of dopamine in his brain, but he is

responsible for increasing his receptiveness to her support. A healthy diet and exercise program increases his potential to produce dopamine and provides the foundation for a loving, happy, and romantic relationship.

2. Declining Interest and Passion

In the beginning of a relationship, a man has plenty of energy, interest, and passion for his partner, but it declines gradually. In a restaurant, you can tell when a man is on a first date; he is giving his full attention while making consistent eye contact with the woman across the table. You can easily tell a married man with his wife; he is usually not making eye contact; he is easily distracted; and the conversation is not as animated.

Eye contact is an indication of dopamine levels. If dopamine levels are normal, a man will effortlessly maintain eye contact. Dopamine increases interest and focus. Wandering eyes are a direct symptom of insufficient dopamine. When a man is in the early stages of a relationship, the newness stimulates his depleted reservoirs of dopamine. Once the newness of the relationship is gone, he requires a much greater stimulation to stay focused unless he has normal levels of dopamine.

Dopamine is the brain hormone of interest. When a man has low dopamine, and the relationship is not new and different, he will quickly lose interest in what his partner has to say. He will feel as if he has heard it before, and he knows where she is going. As a result, it is difficult for him to focus, concentrate, and hear what it is she is saying.

Dopamine is the brain hormone of interest.

With normal dopamine levels, a man doesn't require being on a first date or with a new person to be stimulated. He is automatically more interested in what his wife has to say, just as he was in the beginning of the relationship. With plenty of dopamine, you are not so dependent on new and different experiences.

A man starts out in a relationship with interest, excitement, and enthusiasm, because the relationship is new. Months or years later, his interest wanes. This doesn't mean that he has gradually become dopamine-deficient. Instead, it means that he was dopamine deficient to begin with. When dopamine levels are low, then you need the stimulation of a new relationship to raise dopamine levels and to create energy and attraction.

With very low dopamine levels, a man comes on really strong in the beginning, and then just as quickly his interest disappears. His excitement cannot last. However, with normal dopamine levels, it becomes much easier for men to experience the consistent feelings of interest and attraction as a foundation for making an important commitment.

3. Inattentiveness and Impatience

A man listens to his wife talk about her day and his energy level drops very quickly. He loses his ability to focus like a deflating balloon as she talks beyond two to three minutes. He becomes easily distracted and/or impatient for her to get to the point. This change can actually be measured in his brain. In one minute his prefrontal cortex is active, and then in the next it becomes underactive. This shift occurs with a drop in dopamine.

While listening to a woman share feelings, a man may rapidly lose his ability to focus.

With normal levels of dopamine, a man is able to sustain interest and energy when listening to what his partner has to say. He doesn't need an emergency to occur in order to be energized and motivated. The responsibility of caring for his wife and family is enough to keep his energy up.

4. Impulsiveness

One of the symptoms of low dopamine is impulsiveness. With low dopamine, it is very difficult during a conflict for a man to take a time-out to consider a problem. Either he gets into a big fight without thinking about what he says or does, or he walks away and eventually completely forgets what he was upset about.

At times of conflict, a man with low dopamine finds it more difficult to take a time-out to consider a problem.

One of the symptoms of an underactive prefrontal cortex, which is associated with low dopamine, is the inability to articulate or process inner feelings. Often a man is bothered by something but doesn't really know what it is, nor can he communicate about it. Rather than explore his upset internally and resolve it, he will simply change the subject and do something interesting in order to forget his upset and feel better.

While this flight or avoidance technique helps him cope with stress, he doesn't necessarily resolve his conflicting thoughts and feelings, and they return and accumulate.

For many men, flight is often the preferred choice, particularly in a loving relationship, because they don't want to fight with the woman they love. If a man doesn't have the opportunity to change the subject or take a time-out, he will then move into a more aggressive stance and fight. Either way, instead of resolving issues, he eventually becomes fed up and stops caring as much.

A man commonly feels that everything is fine in a relationship until his partner begins complaining about him. Then, in an instant, he will remember and be upset by his own list about her. He thinks like this: "Everything is okay from my perspective. But if you are going to complain about me, then I will complain about you. I have even more complaints than you, so don't give me such a hard time." This logic may work for him, but not for her. As a result, she will be even more upset.

When a woman begins to complain, a man will
often pull out an even longer list.

If a man has normal dopamine levels, he is able to take a time-out and reflect on his thoughts and feelings when situations upset him. Rather than retaliate, he has the inner control to reflect on why the conflict occurred and then determine what he can do in present time to solve the problem. Dopamine motivates a man to find a solution rather than dwell on the problem.

5. Forgetfulness

A man says he will call after a romantic encounter and then he doesn't. He forgets to do what he intended to do, because after an intimate encounter, dopamine levels drop temporarily. His motivation drops, and he simply forgets. A woman doesn't understand this and is often hurt, because after an intimate encounter, her need for connection and memory increases. When his motivation rises again, he remembers, but it is often too late to call, and he doesn't. He may still be interested, but he doesn't want to be criticized for forgetting to call.

When dopamine levels are normal, a man will tend to remember relationship issues and concerns. If he makes a promise, he will easily remember to fulfill it and be motivated to follow through. When dopamine levels are low, he will still remember things, but only those things that promote the production of dopamine, such as a very important business call, a football game, or the solution of a pressing problem at work.

6. Solution Oriented

A man commonly listens to a woman talk about a problem and then wants her to have a solution right away. He becomes impatient and begins offering solutions. Even if he has read my books explaining that often a woman is looking for understanding and not a solution, he will still feel impatient and forget what it is she needs. Once again, he interrupts with solutions. Without enough dopamine, he forgets just to listen and feels a strong urge to interrupt and give a solution.

With normal dopamine levels and an understanding of what women require, he will be able to listen to her without feeling an urgent need to solve her problem or talk her out of feeling upset. With enough insight, he will have the energy and motivation to listen patiently and compassionately and even ask more questions.

7. Emotional Unavailability

When dopamine levels are low, at the end of his workday, a man goes to his cave but is too tired to come out. As soon as he gets home, he is in no shape to interact. He needs time be on his own without feeling the pressure to be there for someone else. Cave time is time for himself.

After reading *Men Are from Mars,* many women learned not to take his cave time personally. When a man withdraws into his cave, it doesn't mean he doesn't care about her. Instead it is just an expression of his need to be on his own for a while to "take his space." After benefiting from this insight, women then ask, How long does he have to stay in the cave?

When he withdraws into his cave, it doesn't mean he doesn't care about her.

There is no set answer. He stays in the cave as long as it takes. This question is like asking, How long does a woman have to be in a bad mood? or How long does a woman need to talk about her day or her issues? The answer is, As long as it takes. The biggest problem in relationships today is that many men don't make enough dopamine to get out of the cave, and many women don't make enough serotonin to feel fully heard or supported.

The good news is that a man with normal dopamine levels needs much less time in the cave, and he can easily choose when to take that alone time. With adequate dopamine, he is able much of the time to come home and to devote some special time to his wife and children and then take his cave time later.

When women have adequate levels of serotonin, their need to discuss issues goes down dramatically. Within a much shorter period of time, she can get the support she needs to stimulate healthy levels of brain chemicals and hormones. She also doesn't feel the urge to share it all with him. She can easily vent most of her frustrations with other girlfriends and primarily share her warm and friendly feelings with him.

When women have adequate levels of serotonin, their need to discuss issues goes down dramatically.

To stimulate healthy brain chemistry and feel-good hormones in his wife, I suggest that a man devote a good twenty minutes to his wife at least four days a week. This means that before he goes to his cave, he takes time to notice her, ask her about her day, listen and ask more questions, share a little about his day, say nice things to her, give her a hug, be affectionate, and offer to help her with whatever she is doing. These behaviors will stimulate healthy Venusian hormones in her, which in turn will stimulate his dopamine levels.

Devote twenty minutes to a woman when you get home, and she will greatly appreciate you.

Even with adequate amounts of dopamine, a man will still need his cave time, but it will not cause him to be emotionally or physically unavailable for long periods of time. With adequate levels of serotonin, a woman will still need to talk in order to feel and enjoy a connection with her partner. The difference is that it doesn't take as long, and she will feel more satisfied with the outcome. Talking about her day should make a Venusian feel much better. If it doesn't, then either he is not listening or she has low levels of serotonin. Usually both tend to be the case.

8. Tunnel Vision

When dopamine levels are too low, a man focuses on the big problems to solve but overlooks little problems. With his tunnel vision, he can give his attention only to the big fires to put out and ignores, minimizes, overlooks, or dismisses the little problems. Even if they are pointed out to him, he has no energy or attention to solve them. At stressful times, when dopamine production is limited, he can consider only one thing at a time. To interrupt him or ask him to change his focus creates immediate frustration, irritation, and annoyance.

With healthy dopamine levels, a man will still tend to focus on one thing at a time, but he is much more flexible. He can easily shift his attention from big problems to little problems. He is not so cranky when it comes to changed plans or when he is asked to do something different from what he was planning to do. A man will always question if an action is important enough to warrant his attention, but with normal dopamine levels he can be much more compassionate and friendly while considering his options.

9. Boredom and Addictions

With low levels of dopamine, a man is bored with most normal life experiences. To escape this boredom, he will develop addictive tendencies. Almost all addictive behaviors and substance abuse are associated with and are symptoms of extreme low dopamine syndrome. Young boys who don't have access to alcohol, smoking, and drugs will tend to become addicted to sports or video games.

In a marriage, when the security of love becomes comfortable or too routine, a man takes his partner's love and support for granted and loses his feelings of passion. To feel excitement and enthusiasm, he requires excess or extreme stimulation from addictive substances or addictive behaviors.

With low levels of dopamine, a man is bored with most normal life experiences.

Common addictive substances other than drugs are refined sugar, alcohol, cigarettes, and coffee. Common addictive behaviors are overworking, oversleeping, overexercising, focusing too much on sex, excessive TV watching, and too much interest in pornography, to name a few. Sometimes this person doesn't even recognize that he is bored because he simply relies on his addiction to stimulate interest, energy, and pleasure.

When healthy dopamine levels are balanced by normal serotonin levels, all addictive cravings literally go away. When a man's brain is balanced, the normal stimulation from life's challenges is enough to keep him interested and motivated. To experience joy and pleasure, he is not dependent on excess stimulation.

10. Needing Space and Distance

After sex, he will fall asleep right away or suddenly want more space or distance. This doesn't mean in any way that his feelings for her have changed. It just means that he needs to get away to regain his energy and pleasure in life. Being on his own again stimulates increased dopamine, which then gives him more energy.

Autonomy stimulates the production of dopamine.

With healthy brain chemistry, a man doesn't feel the urge to get away right after an experience of intimacy. He enjoys a time of closeness and connection before he feels a normal return to a sense of independence and distance.

Men will always feel an urge to get close and then pull away. Dopamine levels in the brain are associated with the production of the hormone testosterone. When testosterone levels rise, a man's desire to get close increases. Testosterone stimulates the in-and-out urge, and men have much higher levels of testosterone than women. With higher levels of dopamine, testosterone levels are consistent, and this urge to get close and then pull away is more gradual and less extreme. With normal levels of dopamine and testosterone, he doesn't have to climax right away if he is aroused, and he doesn't withdraw so quickly after climax.

11. Inconsistency

When a man has low dopamine, he comes on really strong with great interest and romance in the beginning and then pulls back. Each time he gets close, he backs off. It is hard for his Venusian partner to interpret his feelings because they are so inconsistent. One day he can't live without her and the next he wants to end the relationship. Without understanding this tendency, a woman can easily feel jerked around and confused.

Can't live with them and can't live without them is a classic low dopamine experience.

Often this pattern is misinterpreted to be a fear of intimacy. Generally speaking, if a woman exhibits this inconsistency, it is the symptom of a fear of intimacy caused by some unresolved past issue. If a man exhibits this tendency, it may just disappear by increasing his dopamine levels.

When a man pulls back, it is most often a biological hormonal urge to be on his own. When dopamine levels drop, this urge will be exaggerated. He easily feels smothered in a relationship and has to get away. If a woman is too controlling or mothering, a man, even one with healthy levels of dopamine, will still feel smothered and want to get away. Most men resist being controlled, but lower dopamine has the effect of making a man more sensitive to being controlled by another.

12. Loss of Attraction

A husband loves his wife, but after a few years of marriage, he is not turned on by her the way he was in the beginning. He loves her, but there is less or even no chemistry. Instead of growing in passion as his love grows, his sexual interest declines. When he sees a new and different woman, he may become interested in sex again.

The loss of chemistry in a marriage is not a sign that a man doesn't love his wife.

Unless a man learns to control his urges, he will desire to have affairs. It can be very tempting suddenly to feel alive in the presence of another woman, when at home this feeling is completely missing. This surge of pleasure is similar to having a meal after fasting for several days. It can be very exaggerated and intense. The irony here is that it has nothing to do with love. He will love his wife but be turned on to a complete stranger.

These powerful urges are easily controlled when a man is turned on to his partner and sexually satisfied at home. In a loving relationship, the production of dopamine is fundamental to sustain the chemistry of passion and lasting romance. If a person lacks healthy dopamine levels, getting to know another and living in a routine together can kill passion.

If a person lacks healthy dopamine levels, getting to know another and living in a routine together can kill passion.

With healthy levels of dopamine, a man is still attracted to other women, but because he is also attracted to his wife, he is not tempted to stray. It is a good thing that a man is attracted to other women—this keeps him young and vital. Men are supposed to be attracted to women. By practicing good communication skills, a man can also sustain this primary attraction to his partner.

Having said this, a man can also be rude and insensitive to his partner if he stares at another woman. My wife tells me, "It's okay to look, John, but don't drool." If I do happen to look too long, she just playfully elbows me, and I respond as if awakened from a trance. I quickly send a little extra attention and affection her way.

"It's okay to look at women, just don't drool."

Generally speaking, it is hard for a woman to understand this point instinctively. For her, sexual attraction is not so automatic. She is generally not turned on to a person unless she is interested in having a relationship. Before the urge for sex appears, she needs to feel more of an emotional bond.

UNDERRESPONSIVENESS TO THE NEEDS OF OTHERS

In each of these examples, you can see the theme of ADD and ADHD, but applied to an adult man and his patterns of relating. From a counselor's perspective, a mother's complaints about her ADD or ADHD son are very similar to a woman's complaints about grown men. In both cases, there is a loss of motivation, energy, and patience associated with inattentiveness, hyperactivity, and impulsiveness.

The bottom line of this condition when applied to relationships is best summarized as an *underresponsiveness to the needs of others*. In the beginning of a relationship, even with low dopamine levels, a man is eager to please a woman because the challenge of winning her stimulates adequate levels of dopamine.

Take away the challenge, and dopamine levels drop. Add routine and domesticity, and it drops even more, even when there is a lot of love.

With low dopamine levels, a man is much more eager to please, but only in the beginning of a relationship.

When this man comes home, he thinks he is just tired from working so much. The truth is, he is experiencing low dopamine syndrome. He has energy at work because there is enough risk, challenge, and competition to stimulate dopamine, but at home there is comfort, harmony, and routine. He begins to relax, and because he is dopamine-deficient, he doesn't have any energy without stimulation.

It is not his job that makes him tired. It is low dopamine. If he was single again and starting a new relationship, he would suddenly have plenty of energy after work. Active in the pursuit of finding love, he would suddenly have energy and motivation. As long as he was challenged, he would attentively and actively respond to the different needs of his new partner.

Once he has met her needs and the relationship is secure, his dopamine levels drop, and he becomes underresponsive to her needs. This means he still cares, but he doesn't have the energy to respond to her needs. He has unconsciously budgeted his energy to do the most important things and resists doing the little stuff.

Doing the little stuff is what creates in a woman the feelings of romance and support. It is a man's attention to the little things that stimulates the chemistry of health, happiness, and lasting romance for a woman. In the next chapter, we explore the importance of serotonin in a woman's brain and the many symptoms of low serotonin syndrome that are commonly experienced by millions of women.

4

SEROTONIN IS FROM VENUS

In the West, there is an epidemic of serotonin deficiency in women. Millions of women take such psychoactive medications as Prozac to stimulate the benefits of normal serotonin production. Millions more experience the same symptoms of low serotonin but to a lesser degree. Many of these symptoms are so common that they have come to be viewed over the past thirty years as normal symptoms for women to experience. Various degrees of PMS, feelings of being overwhelmed, overweight, dissatisfaction in relationships, occasional depression, not enough romance, and hot flashes are all considered a normal part of being a woman. They are certainly common, but they are not symptoms of normal health.

In most cases, these unfortunate symptoms are the direct result of a woman's diet and exercise routine. A deficiency in serotonin-producing foods and nutrients results in a host of specific undesirable symptoms for women. Recent research reveals that men synthesize serotonin faster than women and then store twice as much. Most of our serotonin is produced in the morning hours. Without enough production in the morning, a woman can easily run low. While men clearly suffer from the many symptoms of low levels of dopamine, women suffer from low levels of serotonin. Serotonin issues are definitely from Venus.

Low serotonin levels also dramatically affect romantic relationships. Practically every difference between men and women that frustrates men is exaggerated by low serotonin production. Most qualities and characteristics that men love about women are enriched with normal serotonin levels. As a woman begins to produce normal levels of serotonin, not only does she become more desirable to a man, but she experiences sustained health and happiness.

Most women do not need medications. Instead they need a better breakfast to produce normal levels of serotonin in the morning. An adequate production of serotonin in the morning can last throughout the day. When the sun sets, the pineal gland can then convert the remaining serotonin into sufficient melatonin for a good night's sleep. The pineal gland is located in the center of the brain. The pineal gland is directly responsible for the production of serotonin throughout the day and melatonin at night. Without enough melatonin, people find it difficult to get a good night's sleep.

The pineal gland converts extra serotonin into melatonin for a good night's sleep.

Without the right balance of nutrients, particularly at breakfast, a woman will continue to suffer the symptoms of low serotonin throughout her day and even through the night. When these symptoms are extreme, women are motivated to take medications. This condition can be corrected for most women with a diet and exercise program designed to produce more serotonin. Men may also suffer similar symptoms of low serotonin, but this is less common and is usually complicated by low levels of dopamine.

SYMPTOMS OF LOW LEVELS OF SEROTONIN

Serotonin is the neurotransmitter in the brain responsible for the feelings of comfort, satisfaction, contentment, happiness, relaxation, and optimism. Without enough serotonin in her brain, no matter what the circumstances are in her life, a woman will often feel a range of emotions, from being overwhelmed, worried, anxious, regretful, sorrowful, to distressed, resentful, or rigid. Certainly a man may experience drops in his serotonin levels, but nothing like a woman's. When dopamine levels drop, men suffer a sudden decrease in tenderness, understanding, and respect for others. When serotonin levels drop, women suffer from lessened trust, acceptance, and appreciation.

Serotonin gives us the feelings of comfort, happiness, relaxation, and optimism.

The production of serotonin is primarily stimulated by the quality of our relationships. Opportunities to communicate, cooperate, and collaborate in her relationships maximize a woman's production of serotonin. With low levels of serotonin, a woman tends to depend too much on her relationships to stimulate enough of this feel-good hormone. With normal, healthy levels, she is still dependent on the quality of her relationships to stimulate feelings of well-being and optimism, but she is not overly dependent, demanding, or needy. If her levels of serotonin production are low, then no matter how supportive her relationships are, the support will never be enough.

With low levels of serotonin, a woman tends to depend too much on her relationships for happiness.

This is the most common reason women decide to see a counselor. They feel they are not getting enough support in their relationships. If they are not in a relationship, they often feel there are not enough good men available in their circle of friends. Though their complaints may be true to some degree, their conclusions and emotional reactions are complicated and intensified by the inability to produce enough serotonin. In most cases, these symptoms of low levels of serotonin may be the result of a nutritionally deficient diet.

A woman with low levels of serotonin will seek out counseling because talking with someone who cares and is friendly toward her will stimulate the production of serotonin in her brain. To the extent her serotonin levels are low, she will feel a greater need to talk. For some women, less serotonin in the brain means a greater need to talk. The lack of optimism related to low levels of serotonin prevents other women from talking, because they think no one will understand or it will not help.

For some women, less serotonin in the brain means a greater need to talk.

Even if a woman has plenty of opportunities to communicate, cooperate, and collaborate in her life, when her serotonin levels are low, a loving husband who does his best to listen will not be enough. Without the physiological fuel to produce serotonin, a woman will not be satisfied by any amount of talking or romance. She will feel something is missing, and she is right; her brain is not producing enough serotonin.

Without the physiological fuel to produce serotonin, a woman will not be satisfied by any amount of talking or romance.

Millions of women seek out counselors every day to listen to a one-sided conversation for fifty minutes in an attempt to generate enough serotonin to feel good. Though this can be very productive, it doesn't solve a woman's real problem. To complement her therapy, she needs to provide her body with the nutrients necessary to produce more serotonin.

Talking with someone who cares stimulates the production of serotonin.

We need to understand why women depend on counseling so much. Unless it is primarily educational or directed at resolving a past traumatic issue or a current issue, talking to a therapist is really just an expensive replacement for eating a healthy breakfast.

Talking to a therapist can sometimes be an expensive replacement for eating a healthy breakfast.

In some cases, counseling can make a woman's problem worse. She gets relief from the serotonin production that comes from talking and having someone agree with everything she says, but she becomes more intolerant when her husband doesn't. She expects him to be like her therapist and just listen to her. She doesn't realize that she has to listen to him as well. When he wants to be heard or he disagrees, she mistakenly concludes she can't get what she needs.

Even when therapy is effective, the results are often not sustained, because the daily diet doesn't provide the raw material necessary to produce enough serotonin. Starting each day with a serotonin-producing exercise routine and breakfast lessens a woman's need for therapy and increases the possibility of lasting benefits. Let's explore some symptoms of serotonin deficiency syndrome.

1. Temporary Amnesia

One of the most important things a man needs to understand about his wife while they are traveling is the importance of regular food to sustain blood sugar and to produce serotonin. When blood sugar drops, so does the production of serotonin. When a woman is hungry, it is often a sign her blood sugar has dropped. If she says, "Let's look for a restaurant," he needs to interpret this request correctly. It doesn't mean, "Let's casually take twenty or thirty minutes to find food." It means, "Do it now."

Women are more dependent on regular food intake to keep blood sugar up and sustain the production of serotonin. This regular need for food becomes even more important when a woman doesn't start her day with a lot of serotonin production.

If she indicates that she needs food, he should treat it like a code blue alert. In hospitals, when someone has a heart attack, he needs urgent attention to stay alive. This need for urgent care and maximum concern is indicated by the term *code blue*. When a wife or daughter needs to eat, a man needs to hear this as a code blue alert. Get her food right away.

When a wife or daughter needs to eat, a man needs to get her food right away.

If a woman doesn't eat right away when she feels hunger, her blood sugar and serotonin levels will drop within a few minutes. When this occurs, she is no longer the woman he married. For this brief period of time, she will experience temporary amnesia and forget any good thing he has ever done.

When blood sugar drops, a woman experiences temporary amnesia and forgets every good thing a man has ever done.

This amnesia can occur whenever blood sugar drops. This is not the time to argue with her or remind her of all the reasons you are a great guy.

If she says you are always late, don't remind her of the times when you have been on time.

If she says she does everything, don't point out to her that you do a lot, too.

If she says you are not romantic or loving anymore, don't point out the last time you were romantic.

If she looks at you as if you are a complete disappointment to her, don't take it personally—let it go. Trust that this cloud will pass, and once again the sun will shine.

**When a woman's blood sugar drops,
trust that this cloud will pass, and once again
the sun will shine.**

Realize that when a woman's blood sugar drops, she will take poetic license while expressing her feelings. Don't take what she says literally and don't argue. Whatever she says, just listen and get food.

Solve the real problem. Get food and do your best not to say anything. By listening, you will help stimulate a rise in her serotonin levels until you can get her some food. With the right fuel, she will suddenly be back to the woman who loves you and remembers what a great guy you are.

2. Sudden Mood Changes

Men must understand the link between blood sugar, serotonin, and sudden mood swings. Sugar feeds the brain. When blood sugar levels drop, the brain's production of serotonin stops, and a woman's mood sinks. With this insight, a man can show his support by listening and getting food and not taking a woman's words, feelings, and attitudes personally. He will often get emotionally bruised and react defensively when he doesn't understand the many reasons for her sudden attitude change. Some experts estimate that more than 75 percent of women experience daily blood sugar drops. In Chapter 11, we will explore in much greater detail why women experience low blood sugar and what they can do to avoid this imbalance.

A woman's mood can change very quickly. One minute she is appreciating and enjoying a man, and the next she is emotionally upset, doubting him and asking him a lot of questions. He feels she is rejecting him or treating him like someone who doesn't love, care for, and support her. One minute he is a great guy, and the next she looks at him as if he is a big zero!

One minute you are a great guy, and the next she looks at you as if you are a big zero!

Moderate mood swings are normal. They are natural and occur just like the weather changes. Some days are warm, some are cold, some are bright and sunny, while others are overcast or rainy. These changes make life interesting and fulfilling. When serotonin levels are low, these natural mood changes become more sudden and dramatic. Instead of rain, you get hurricanes.

When serotonin levels are low, natural mood changes become more sudden and dramatic.

Even with healthy serotonin levels, a woman's mood will change suddenly. Her feelings rise and fall from positive and then to negative in a wavelike fashion. Women instinctively understand this, but men don't. Men don't have bodies that undergo massive hormonal changes to potentially create a baby every month.

The regular changes in a woman's hormonal balance due to her menstrual cycle are responsible for her ever-changing emotional landscape. For some period of time, her mood rises and she sees everything in a more positive light. She feels a sense of abundance in her life. When that wave reaches its peak, it can go only one direction—down. As her wave begins to drop, a woman becomes more aware of her need to receive more support. If she is not getting enough support in her life, this is when she will feel it. Without adequate serotonin in her brain, she will undergo a dramatic crash.

When her wave crashes, a man mistakenly thinks he has to fix her or solve all her problems. He may conclude that there is nothing he can do to make her happy. He thinks she will never be happy unless all her problems get solved. He feels defeated and his dopamine levels drop. He suddenly has little energy or interest in what she is saying.

By remembering how he can help, he can keep his dopamine levels elevated to stay focused and supportive. Once her emotional wave hits bottom, her mood will automatically swing to positive again. With a balanced diet and an exercise plan to facilitate her changing hormonal levels, her emotional wave can be like a gentle hill instead of jagged mountain peaks and valleys.

3. Increased Neediness

From an evolutionary point of view, a woman's changing emotional needs make sense. When her serotonin levels are high, a woman has less need for relationships. She is more autonomous. When her estrogen levels drop at the time of ovulation, her serotonin levels also drop. This drop increases her need for relationships. On a hormonal level, she is more likely to create communication, cooperation, and collaboration in her relationships.

At this time of lower serotonin levels, her body is preparing to get pregnant, and her need for relationships increases. When she is ovulating, her brain is hardwired to seek out love and support. From an evolutionary perspective, this desire for love and support increases her chances of getting pregnant. She suddenly appreciates more potential romantic partners.

When a woman is ovulating, her needs in her
relationships increase.

This pattern is efficient unless a woman already has significantly low levels of serotonin. Instead of experiencing a slight drop in serotonin to stimulate a greater need for relationships, she suffers from increased neediness. With a sudden shift in hormones, she may feel abandoned and hopeless and then react defensively with feelings of annoyance, irritation, and indifference. These symptoms are often labeled PMS (premenstrual syndrome). At these times, when her wave crashes, talking about her feelings makes her serotonin levels rise, and she begins to feel better.

With a sudden shift in hormones, a woman may feel abandoned and hopeless.

With this insight, a man may find it easier to give up trying to solve her problems, lecture her, or explain to her why she shouldn't be upset about something. Instead, he can wisely listen, ask questions, and give her wave a chance to fall gracefully and then rise back up. Then she will begin to brighten up.

By listening, caring, and trying to be a friend at these times, a man will assist her brain in producing serotonin. This increased production of serotonin will enable her to hit bottom faster and then come back up into a good mood. Understanding what is actually happening allows a man to be more patient, because he now knows it may get worse before it gets better.

A wise man knows it may get worse before it gets better.

If a woman is suffering from low serotonin syndrome because her diet is deficient in nutrients, no amount of love and support from her partner will ever be enough. A wise woman recognizes that her diet, exercise routine, and lifestyle choices are just as important as the love and support she can get in a romantic relationship.

Unless she accepts the importance of her diet and exercise, she will conclude that her partner is incapable of giving her enough support at times of disappointment or unhappiness. Rather than enjoy and appreciate what he has to offer, she will focus on what she is not getting. When her brain chemistry is healthy, her neediness will lessen dramatically.

4. Looking for Love in All the Wrong Places

Giving of ourselves in a relationship is the one behavior that most dramatically stimulates the production of serotonin. When serotonin levels are healthy, a woman will feel an urge to give to someone who has the potential to give back or to someone who has already given her support. This healthy giving response is based on reciprocity. She gives, but she also receives back. She receives, and then she gives back. This balance of giving and receiving provides fulfillment in relationships.

A balance of giving and receiving provides fulfillment in relationships.

If a woman already has an abundance of support in her life, her fulfillment can rise to an even higher level. She can give to those who cannot give back to her. This unconditional giving is like giving to a charity. It is giving freely without the need to receive anything in return.

Charitable giving provides the highest fulfillment. It is giving without any expectation that one will receive back. On a biochemical level, this kind of unconditional giving produces a rush of the hormone oxytocin, and this in turn stimulates more serotonin. (Oxytocin is the hormone of well-being on Venus. We will explore this hormone in much greater detail in Chapter 6.) By giving without expecting a return, you can always get an immediate dose of serotonin.

Giving without expectations produces maximum serotonin.

To experience the relief of increased serotonin, a woman may give of herself without the expectation of return. Instead of waiting to give to someone who can return her support, she is attracted to situations, circumstances, and people unable to return her support. To gain immediate serotonin relief, she will look for love in all the wrong places.

After giving and giving, one morning she wakes up and feels completely empty from giving too much. Giving to a charity makes you feel really good, but it is not a good thing if you have to go into debt. On the other hand, if your needs are already being met, you can afford the luxury of giving to those who cannot return your support.

Without enough serotonin, some women consistently give where they cannot get back and reject opportunities to receive from those who really have something to give. Even if someone wants to give, these women don't open up to receive. They are so busy trying to earn love in all the wrong places that they cannot relax enough to receive help. Fortunately, this can change.

By establishing healthy levels of serotonin, a woman is more likely to be attracted to people and situations with the potential to give her more support. When she is not dependent on giving without getting back to feel good, she can relax and receive more. When this happens, her awareness expands to recognize the tremendous support already available in her life.

5. Resentment Flu

What always follows giving too much is resentment. When a woman gives too much, she will inevitably begin to expect, demand, or require more in return. When she doesn't get back what she is giving, she will begin to feel resentment. This resentment may even become chronic, particularly when her brain is not producing enough serotonin.

Hurt and resentment can be observed in the brain with modern technology as increased activity in the limbic system of the brain. When a man remembers being hurt, blood flows to the limbic system of the brain, which governs emotions.

When a woman remembers being hurt, *eight times* more blood flows to the limbic system. This increased emotional sensitivity as indicated by increased blood flow in women is normal and healthy.

Women are designed to be more emotionally vulnerable and sensitive.

In a healthy brain, once the limbic system gets overactivated, serotonin is stimulated and washes over the limbic system, allowing it to relax. A woman may be hurt, but she can easily bounce back with forgiveness, acceptance, understanding, and trust. When she does not produce enough serotonin in her brain, the limbic system remains overactive and doesn't relax. Her hurt feelings become chronic and eventually turn into resentment, confusion, and mistrust.

The limbic system in the brain is like a filter through which you interpret the events of the day. The limbic system determines whether you see the glass as half full or half empty. Brain research on women with PMS symptoms reveals that a few days before the onset of menstruation, the deep limbic system becomes inflamed or overactive.

Some of the symptoms of an overactive limbic system are:

- Moodiness, irritability, and depression
- Increased negative thinking
- Negative anticipation of events
- Decreased motivation to give
- Strong negative emotions
- Overeating
- Difficulty sleeping
- Decreased or increased sexual interest

When a woman doesn't have enough serotonin, her limbic system may remain overactive. Resentment is not only sustained but increases over time. This chronic resentment is a sickness. It is like getting the flu. When you get the flu, there is little you can do but ride it out and nurture yourself with lots of water, minerals, and rest. Likewise in relationships, when a woman catches resentment flu from giving too much, she needs to stop giving to others and start giving to herself. This healthy shift is hard to make if she is low in serotonin.

Chronic resentment is a sickness like the flu.

The behavior cure for chronic resentment is to stop giving in relationships from which you are not getting back and to let go of all your expectations for a while. Focus on giving where you can get back. First give to yourself, and then give to friends who can and will give back to you.

When you feel resentment flu, it is not the time for charitable giving. It may feel good to give, but when you come back to your relationship, you will experience even more resentment. At times of resentment, you have to make sure you receive what you need from where it is easily available. Even though you may love giving, give to yourself for a while.

**When you feel resentment flu,
it is not the time for charitable giving.**

This shift is different from withholding your love. When you go to the Bahamas or Hawaii on vacation, you are not rejecting your home. You are simply taking time off somewhere to nurture yourself so that you can return home rejuvenated and more fully appreciative of where you live. It is a choice to serve and nurture your personal needs.

Often in relationships, women feel guilty making a choice to nurture their own needs. They believe that to get their needs met, they must give to others. When they are not getting what they need, the last thing they would instinctively do is to stop giving. Instead of giving to themselves, women will continue giving to others and complain that they are not getting back. This is like canceling a vacation and choosing to stay home but complaining the whole time that she hasn't taken a vacation!

In a relationship, one of the worst things a woman can do to herself and to others is to give only in her actions, not from an open heart. Action produces dopamine, but unless she is giving from an open heart in the spirit of loving communication, cooperation, and collaboration, she will inhibit the production of serotonin, and her resentment will just increase.

When a woman does the right thing but without an open heart, it only fuels her resentment.

Ironically, when a man is feeling resentful or unloving, the best thing for him is to perform some action in the service of others. Even if he doesn't feel very loving and he doesn't really feel like doing it, by doing the right thing in service of another, a man can raise his testosterone levels, which in turn raises his dopamine levels. As his Martian hormones begin to rise, he will start feeling more motivated to be loving, helpful, and compassionate. Instead of just doing the right thing, he will *feel* like doing it as well.

For a man, the old-fashioned notion of "just do the right thing" regardless of how he feels will produce dopamine, and he will start to experience greater pleasure, energy, and motivation. Automatically he feels more loving and supportive. He does not need more serotonin to generate feelings of love. Instead, he needs more dopamine to remember and tap into the love he already feels.

Increasing a woman's dopamine levels by doing the right thing does not increase her serotonin levels. Women generally have plenty of dopamine and are already motivated to do the right thing. That is why a woman keeps giving in service to others instead of to herself. When she feels resentful, she first needs to do something for herself to feel good, and then doing the right thing in the service of others will make her feel even better.

Being married to a partner who does not meet her emotional

needs is often a part of the low serotonin cycle. After years of not getting what she needs in a relationship, a woman may feel resentment and forget the reasons she fell in love. At such times, she will begin to doubt her partner and conclude he doesn't love her. This may be true, but most often it is not.

**A woman may feel resentful
and forget the reasons she fell in love.**

Like having a toothache, when a woman has the resentment flu, she may find it hard to think loving thoughts or be nice. Although she may love her partner and continue to do loving things for him, she will be unable to feel true appreciation for him. Instead of delighting in the many things he does provide for her, she will focus or even obsess on how much *she* does and how little he does.

When a woman gets resentment flu, she can't feel loving just by trying. She can do loving things, but her heart is not open. With a closed heart she begins to keep score, and he always ends up short. If the score is sixty points for her good deeds and twenty points for his good deeds, she subtracts twenty from sixty and comes up with a new score: forty to zero. At these times she actually feels as if he does nothing for her. This is the symptom of resentment flu.

No one with a toothache can be nice and friendly.

After years of resentment flu, the malady may eventually turn into resentment pneumonia. At this point, she will mistakenly think she married the wrong man and consider divorce. She is certainly not getting what she needs in her marriage, but this doesn't mean that she couldn't get what she needs. Just finding the right person for you doesn't ensure that you will get what you need. How much and what you get in a relationship has less to do with your partner and more to do with the way you react and respond to that person.

> What you get in a relationship has less to do with
> your partner and more to do with the way you
> react and respond to that person.

When women think about getting a divorce, the most common message I hear is "I give and give and I don't get back what I need." Understanding resentment flu can begin to solve this problem. Instead of leaving their partners to repeat the pattern, women learn a different way of giving. Instead of giving all the time and hoping to get back, these women learn to give to themselves.

> In counseling sessions, what I hear over
> and over is "I give and give and I don't
> get back what I need."

With this new insight, women can give themselves permission to stop sacrificing for their partners and start doing what they would enjoy doing. Instead of expecting their partners to make them happy and feeling obligated to meet all their partners' needs, they begin giving for themselves as well.

It is unhealthy to give it all to your spouse and then expect him to meet all your needs. The solution in relationships is to do what you need to do so that you get the emotional support you need, and then you can truly give without expectations for your spouse and children. This kind of relationship is much more fulfilling.

6. Unrealistic Expectations

Women assume that because men know so much about the world and the way things work that they must also know the way women think and feel. This is an unrealistic expectation. Just because a man loves a woman doesn't mean he will behave or give love the way a woman in love does. Men want to make women happy; they just don't understand what women need most.

The truth is, most men don't even have a clue. Once they begin to find out, it will still take many years before they can really get a handle on what a woman's unique needs are. Without an understanding of how different men and women are, a woman unnecessarily blames her partner. She concludes that he *does* know better. She then feels hurt or unsupported because he doesn't care enough to do the things that would matter most for her. This blaming attitude not only pushes men away but also reinforces her mistaken belief that she is not loved.

Normal levels of serotonin relax the brain. Low levels of serotonin are linked to an overactive cingulate system in the brain. The cingulate system is deep in the middle of the brain running from front to back. It has to do with feeling safe and secure and gives us the ability to go with the flow and adapt to change. One of the symptoms of an overactive cingulate system in the brain is what scientists call cognitive inflexibility. In simple terms, this means that a person is unable to shift gears and let go of an expectation.

Low serotonin results in cognitive inflexibility, or the inability to shift gears and let go of an expectation or belief.

If someone disappoints us, the cingulate system in the brain allows us to adjust to the new situation with insight and make the best of it. Cognitive inflexibility inhibits a person's ability to go with the flow and simply accept what life has to offer. It also creates an urgency for things to be done now. Not later, but now!

These tendencies are magnified in a woman's romantic relationships. The more she gives to someone in an intimate relationship, the more inflexible she will become when she doesn't get what she expects.

If a stranger is late, she can be graceful, forgiving, and

understanding, but when it is someone to whom she has been giving a lot, she becomes more inflexible. Her rationale is "I do all this for you, you *should* do that for me."

In the beginning of a relationship, even with low levels of serotonin, a woman can be forgiving of her partner's mistakes and imperfections. In the beginning, she does not expect anything from him. As she does things for him, her expectations of what she should get in return go up. With cognitive inflexibility she finds it hard to let go of her expectations and be happy with what she gets.

With cognitive inflexibility we find it hard to be happy with what we get in life.

As the relationship unfolds, instead of growing to accept her partner more, she holds on to the pain of unfulfilled expectations and feels increasingly disappointed and unforgiving of his mistakes. After many years of marriage and cognitive inflexibility, a woman will chronically predict that she will not get what she wants. When her serotonin levels increase, her overactive cingulate system can relax, and healthy optimism is restored. Instead of holding on to what happened in the past, she becomes more optimistic. She begins predicting and appreciating what she can get instead of what she won't get.

The cingulate system of the brain allows us to shift our priorities as situations change. When the cingulate system is dysfunctional, we have a tendency to get locked into our expectations of how life should be. As a result, we resist change. This can show up in a variety of ways, from being upset if plans change at the last minute to requiring our environment always to be neat and orderly. Certainly, some of this is normal and determined by temperament or personality, but when it becomes excessive, it is associated with an overactive cingulate system and/or low serotonin levels.

Other symptoms associated with an overactive cingulate system are:

- Excessive worrying (she worries for the whole family)
- Holding on to hurts from the past (she remembers only his mistakes)
- Getting stuck on negative thoughts
- Wanting things now or in a particular manner
- Automatic resistance to change
- Inability to forgive and forget easily

If there is an expectation or plan, an overactive cingulate system requires that we stick to it. A woman will exhibit these tendencies when her serotonin levels are low.

By giving too much to her partner and expecting too much in return, a woman can easily sabotage the success of her relationship. With the epidemic levels of low dopamine in men and low serotonin in women, it is a miracle that only 50 percent of marriages end in divorce. By expecting too much from a man, a woman unknowingly creates an obstacle to receiving his support.

By expecting too much from a man, women unknowingly sabotage their romantic relationships.

Men are motivated to give more when what they do give is appreciated. If a woman responds with the feeling that he is not giving enough, he will automatically begin to give less. When a woman has resentment flu, she is unable to appreciate his attempts to make things better. Inevitably, he will give less and less and then give up.

Appreciation for his efforts is a reward for his efforts. When a man knows he will get a reward for something, his dopamine levels rise and he is more motivated to give. A man is most excited and motivated when he feels he can make a difference. When a woman catches resentment flu, he will often give up giving, because what he does doesn't seem to make a difference. Nothing he says or does can make her happy.

7. Sabotaging Her Relationships

Women will often point out to me that they didn't always have resentment flu. They wonder why men give more when women were feeling their appreciation for their men. The answer to this question points out another difference. Men are most motivated when you ask for what you want. Unless you ask for more, he assumes that you are getting what you want. This is a delicate issue, because if you ask for too much, he assumes you don't appreciate what he has given. The safe solution is to ask for more in small increments.

Unless you ask for more, a man assumes that you are getting what you want.

When a woman expresses her love and appreciation by giving more, a man's motivation to give back can be blocked because he gets the message that he has already given enough. Men tend to give the most when they feel needed. If she is not asking for his support, he mistakenly concludes that he is already doing enough. Every day, millions of women sabotage their relationships by *not* asking for what they want in a language that will motivate a man to respond.

By giving too much to a man, a woman can block a man from giving more.

Women don't readily see how they sabotage their relationships with men, because on Venus, giving more motivates another Venusian to give more in response. When you give to a man, he often assumes that he has already done something to earn your gift. Giving to a man or doing things for him conveys the message that he is already giving enough. It is as if you are saying, "You have done such a great job, now you can rest, relax, and receive back."

To get more in a relationship, a woman needs to give less and appreciate more what he gives. A man's dopamine levels are stimulated when he gets the message that what he provides is good enough *and* he is needed for a specific task.

When a woman can ask a man for more specific support with a tone of appreciation for what she is already getting, her chances of getting what she needs dramatically go up. She needs to be friendly, appreciative, and specific in her request. For example, instead of saying, "We never go out anymore," she could say, "Let's do something special this weekend. Would you make reservations for eating out at El Franio or Roxanne's?"

Men are most motivated when there is a problem they can solve. They are least motivated when they are viewed as the problem. Complaining can zap a man of all his good intentions in a moment. Making specific requests can pull the best from him.

To get more in a relationship, a woman needs to give less and appreciate more what he gives.

Sometimes as I teach women about men, they resist the notion that a man's love for a woman doesn't necessarily motivate him to give. She figures that since she is motivated to give, he should be motivated if he loves her. She doesn't realize that her readiness to give comes from a deficiency of serotonin. When serotonin levels are low, she gets an immediate reward from her brain by giving. He doesn't.

Unless a man anticipates getting a reward for his actions, his brain does not supply the necessary dopamine to sustain motivation. For a man, love is not enough. He needs clear messages that he is needed and appreciated for his brain to produce dopamine, providing him with the energy available to do more. Understanding brain biochemistry makes this difference between Mars and Venus much easier for women to understand.

The same man who would give his life to save his partner because he loves her so much will forget to empty the trash, fall asleep from boredom with too many details in a conversation, or experience sudden brain fog while she is talking about problems that he can do nothing to solve.

8. The Home Improvement Committee

Women with low levels of serotonin are motivated to give more, not just because they are needed, but because giving stimulates missing brain chemicals. When a woman loves a man, to sustain the production of serotonin in her brain, she will feel a need to help him even though he may not be asking for that help. When her levels of serotonin are lower, this tendency becomes magnified. With love in her heart, she forms the home improvement committee and focuses all her attention on changing him.

When men get married, they hope that their partner will not change. Women rejoice because now they can work on changing him. This attempt to improve a man is generally not well received by men. If she wants to improve him, he perceives that he is not accepted the way he is. Acceptance is very important to men. Her attempts to help him are often interpreted as criticism. One of the biggest mistakes a woman makes in a relationship is to offer unsolicited advice.

One of the biggest mistakes a woman makes with a man is to offer unsolicited advice.

The lower a woman's levels of serotonin, the more she searches out ways to give and feel needed. Rather than focus on what *she* needs to feel good, she focuses on how he needs to change. If she takes more time to nurture and improve herself instead of him, not only will she be happier, but he will be more interested in what he can do to please her.

When a woman grows and changes, a man is automatically inspired to change and improve his ways. If she attempts to improve him and he is not directly asking for this kind of support, he will resist change even more. This can kill the passion in a relationship. To grow in love, a man needs to get the message that he can be himself. With this message, he is inspired to be all that he can be. With this support, passion can grow over time rather than dwindle away.

To grow in love, a man needs to get the message that he can be himself.

Instead of trying to help a man, a woman needs to focus more on how she needs his help. Since men generally have higher levels of serotonin, they don't get motivated unless they get a clear message that they are needed. When a man receives the message that a specific action is required, dopamine gets produced in his brain to give him energy and motivation.

Because men have higher levels of serotonin, they are not automatically motivated to give.

This concept is essential to being a man. It is as if every cell in his body follows the Martian rule of behavior: "Do only what you have to do." This conservation of energy is more important to him because his levels of energy are determined by his dopamine levels, and most men have low dopamine, particularly at home.

A woman misinterprets this low energy and increased emphasis on doing only what has to be done as a lack of caring or just plain laziness. From a man's point of view, he is just being efficient. He also thinks he is saving his energy for an emergency. With low dopamine levels throughout his life, he has no idea that he already has the potential to experience endless energy.

From a man's point of view, doing less means conserving energy and being efficient.

When a man has higher levels of dopamine, stimulated by a supportive relationship and a healthy diet and exercise program, he has so much energy that he doesn't have to be so careful with his energy. He has so much dopamine that he is motivated to do things most of the time.

Since men have plenty of serotonin, they do not suffer from such problems as giving too much. As we have discovered, they suffer from a lack of energy and motivation at home. With this insight, a woman can avoid taking his lack of motivation personally. It also gives her permission to ask for more without having to give more.

By learning to give a little less and in turn giving more to herself and her friends, a married woman will find that her husband is more interested in her again. Men are always drawn to those who can, will, and do appreciate what they are offering.

9. Women Who Give Too Much

With lower levels of serotonin, women are driven by feelings of excessive caring, obligation, and responsibility for others. These women feel that they give more than they get in their relationships and lives. In the beginning of relationships, they are happy to give, and later on, that changes. Giving more is fine until others don't respond to her in the same manner. At a certain point, a woman becomes tired of giving and not getting back.

When this occurs, she can either be accountable for her predicament or be a victim. If she chooses to be a victim, she has not received back what she needs. From the perspective of being responsible for the results she gets in life, she has given too much or unfairly expected too much. When women give too much, they will always get less in life.

When women give too much, they will always get less in life.

This situation can be compared to investing in the stock market. If you put all your money in one stock and it goes down, you clearly invested too much. It is a case of putting all your eggs in one basket. In the stock market, this accountability is clear, but that is not always the case in relationships. Most of the time, a woman will tend to blame her partner for not giving back enough, instead of wisely becoming responsible for how much and when she gives of herself.

A wise investor first makes secure investments and then uses extra money to take risks. If he gets a return on his more risky investments, that is an extra perk, but his security comes from a balanced portfolio of conservative stocks, bonds, cash, and real estate.

In a similar manner, we need to invest our time, energy, love, and attention where it will first yield conservative benefits for us. Thinking of others and not of yourself is just as imbalanced and destructive as thinking only of yourself. Women with low serotonin will often give and give until they have nothing left to give. Eventually they become resentful and exhausted.

Thinking of others and not of yourself is just as imbalanced and destructive as thinking only of yourself.

By understanding this pattern, women can release this resentment and choose a more effective approach. By becoming accountable for giving too much, a woman can begin to shift her behaviors to giving in more appropriate ways. High-risk investments are only for those who have a lot of backup money.

Giving without expectations is a luxury for those who already have high serotonin levels.

Becoming accountable for giving too much is a much more enlightened perspective than feeling victimized, but even this perspective is limited. Giving too much is really not the problem. Giving makes us feel good. Giving is a good thing to do! The problem is failing to get what we need.

Finding this balance of giving and receiving can be elusive for women, because regardless of the emotional support they receive in return, they do get the immediate benefits of increased production of serotonin when they give. The lower a woman's serotonin levels, the more relief she will feel by simply giving regardless of what she gets back.

10. Feeling Overwhelmed

Giving too much leads a woman into the most common symptom of low serotonin syndrome: feeling overwhelmed. Women have not always felt overwhelmed. It is a new phenomenon. Just as ADD and ADHD for boys and men have started to emerge in epidemic proportions, so also has the female equivalent emerged. As a counselor for thirty years, I have witnessed the word *overwhelmed* gradually creep into our common vernacular. Instead of saying, "I am unhappy and dissatisfied," women today describe the experience of feeling overwhelmed.

Overwhelmed has a more positive spin, which is also more accurate. If you are simply unhappy, it can easily imply you are not loving enough to appreciate what you have. To be overwhelmed implies that you are so loving that you are trying to give your all. Women do not feel, "There is too much to do, so I don't care." In biochemical terms, if a woman with low serotonin is trying to be loving, she will feel doubtful that she can get everything done. She will feel as if she can't get the support she needs to do what she wishes she could do.

The word *overwhelmed* accurately describes the daily experience of a person experiencing low serotonin levels.

Too much to do and not enough time to do it has become the subject of conversation for millions of women every day. These women make the mistake of thinking their feelings are determined by their stressful lives. But this is just not true. There is no shortage of time. There have always been twenty-four hours in a day, and there always will be. Stress doesn't have to make a person feel overwhelmed, but it will if you have low serotonin levels.

Too much to do and not enough time is the subject of conversation for millions of women every day.

Low serotonin makes you care too much about what other people think. When you care too much, then you feel a compulsion to do it all. When you place too much emphasis on what others think, you don't take the time to discover what you think or what you want. By slowing down and doing things for yourself to discover and enjoy what you like, want, and need for yourself, you can begin to shake the grip of your obsessions.

Low serotonin makes you care too much what other people think.

Feeling overwhelmed is just a mild version of obsessive-compulsive disorder (OCD), which is caused by an overactive brain deficient in serotonin. Instead of relaxing at the end of the day, a woman might spend her evening worrying about what she has to do, what she has not done, what she can't get done, what needs to be done, what will happen if it isn't done, and on and on. As women eat in a way to sustain the production of serotonin, their brains can relax more and the tendency to over-analyze that can permeate a woman's life will begin to disappear. As the brain relaxes, a woman can easily give up her perfectionism and compulsion to please others. Instead, she can live a balanced life of giving to others and giving to herself.

With normal serotonin levels, women are able to relax and to prioritize what needs to be done. One of the symptoms of being overwhelmed is an expanded awareness of so many problems and potential problems that one is paralyzed and doesn't know where to start.

With low serotonin, one will find it hard to make a decision.

The mind is flooded with too many obligations and promises to fulfill for others. With adequate serotonin, the brain can relax and discern what is most important without feeling pressured by other responsibilities.

11. Depression

The most researched symptom of low serotonin syndrome is clinical depression. Tens of millions of women today are diagnosed with depression and are being treated with such psychoactive drugs as Prozac and Zoloft. Statistically, women are two or three times as likely as men to suffer from clinical depression, and four times more likely to suffer from symptoms of seasonal affective disorder (SAD). Millions more go untreated and undiagnosed.

As many as 70 percent of the nation's 30,000 suicides annually can be attributed to undiagnosed depression. More women attempt suicide. With their high dopamine levels, three times as many men actually follow through and commit suicide. For every suicide, hundreds more seriously consider the act. More than 50 million Americans feel debilitated by some form of depression or anxiety every year. The costs of medical care, lost work time, and loss of life associated with depressive disorders are estimated to be in the range of $40 billion annually. Recent research also reveals a direct link between longevity and the ability to avoid depression.

Serotonin is the best-known depression-relieving neurotransmitter. Correct amounts of serotonin can lead to feelings of emotional stability, well-being, personal security, relaxation, calmness, tranquility, and confidence. Low levels of serotonin lead to the many symptoms of depression. These include:

- Chronic distress and despair
- Strong feelings of guilt and regret
- Feelings of isolation, abandonment, and hopelessness
- An overall indifference toward life and relationships
- Inhibited sexual desire

- A numbness or flatness of feeling
- Inability to sleep at night
- Lack of passion or interest
- Resistance to having fun
- An unwillingness to try to make a relationship work
- Chronic fatigue
- Little hunger or excessive hunger

Most of these symptoms of depression are directly related to an overactive limbic system in the brain, which can be relieved by the relaxing influence of adequate production of serotonin. It is so gratifying for me to see these symptoms suddenly disappear without the need for medication in the thousands of people who are already enjoying *The Mars and Venus Diet and Exercise Solution.*

Besides dopamine deficiency in men, one of the main reasons so many relationships and marriages fail is that women are unable to sustain their feelings of happiness and hope in their relationships. A quick review of the above symptoms of depression can explain why men have only one complaint when they are not satisfied in a relationship. A man will almost always complain, "No matter what I do, it is not enough to make her happy." Without the feedback that he is making a difference in a relationship, men find it hard to produce adequate dopamine levels to stay motivated and keep trying.

With a natural means to produce serotonin each day, a woman can begin to create the brain chemistry of health, happiness, and lasting romance. With this support, she can easily give a man the positive messages of appreciation, acceptance, and trust that will stimulate the production of dopamine in him so that he can continue giving his best in their relationship.

12. Obesity and Emotional Eating

Many women avoid or at least minimize feelings of depression by emotional eating. They overeat to soothe their overactive, serotonin-deficient brains. If they are fortunate to be born with more fat cells, these women suffer from weight gain instead of enduring the effects of an overactive brain when blood sugar rises and falls due to an unhealthy diet. This is an advantage, because an obese woman knows that her diet may be killing her.

Women in the normal weight range or moderately overweight women are also dying from an unhealthy diet, but they don't experience physical symptoms until their sickness is in its later stages. Cancer, heart disease, and osteoporosis don't just happen overnight. These diseases may begin twenty years before the symptoms show up. The early warning stages of sickness for lean or moderately overweight women are worrying, obsessing, and all the other, more psychological symptoms of low serotonin.

At least an obese woman knows that her diet may be killing her.

Most women who are not overweight also overeat. A symptom of low serotonin is emotional eating. Emotional eating is eating just to feel comfort, ease, and optimism. Research reveals that *all* obese women are serotonin-deficient.

Research reveals that *all* obese women are serotonin-deficient.

When you have healthy levels of serotonin, you don't eat to feel good. You already feel good, and you eat because you are hungry. When you are hungry, food tastes really good. Even healthful foods like salads and vegetables taste really good.

While some women overgive to produce serotonin, others will overthink (obsess about the negative), and still others will overeat. Some women do all these things. As a matter of fact, most women will turn to junk food to find comfort at times of emotional distress. They medicate their emotional pain with unhealthy food.

There is nothing wrong with using food as your medicine. The problem is that unhealthy women pick the wrong foods.

When the brain is out of balance, you will always crave unhealthy foods. If you are unhappy, you will hunger for foods that will give you momentary happiness and then leave you depleted and more unhappy.

When you begin to balance your brain chemistry, you will naturally eat foods that sustain the production of serotonin. With a knowledge of how to begin producing serotonin, you will be on your way to eliminating any or all of the twelve symptoms of low serotonin syndrome.

Eating a healthy breakfast puts your brain in balance so that you hunger for the right amount of healthier foods. If you skip breakfast or eat an imbalance of nutrients for the rest of the day, you will be out of balance and it will take willpower to keep your diet healthy.

In the Mars and Venus Solution, no willpower is needed. It actually gets in the way. If you eat a breakfast that feeds your brain, you will find that your brain does the rest for you. It effortlessly directs the body to hunger for healthier foods. All you have to do is enjoy eating them.

5

ENDORPHINS ARE FROM HEAVEN

The public awareness of endorphins dramatically increased in the early eighties when masses of people began jogging every day to feel good, lose weight, and achieve better health. The best thing about this movement was the recognition that physical activity and exercise play an enormous role in our sense of well-being and happiness. We learned that jogging produces endorphins in the brain, and suddenly all our worries went down the drain.

Endorphins make us happy and joyful. With a surge of endorphin production in the brain, we feel completely alive, strong, and energized. Unfortunately, the price many joggers pay at midlife and beyond is knee surgeries, arthritis, painful joints, and accelerated aging. Fortunately, there are other ways to produce endorphins.

Jogging or any strenuous exercise can certainly be good for you if you are in shape and your body is designed for that kind of exercise. Some experts, however, point out that only 10 percent of joggers have bodies designed to run for several miles.

How do you know if your body is designed to jog? I would like to say that if you love to jog, then it is right for you, but this is not always the case. The basic rule of thumb is if you are sore the next day, then you are jogging too much.

> The basic rule of thumb is if you are sore the next
> day, then you are exercising or jogging too much.

Jerry Seinfeld did a funny skit about this. He pointed out that personal trainers have you work out to feel really good in your body. After you work out, you feel really sore. When you complain that you don't feel better but actually worse, they say that is why you have to exercise more; that when you get in shape, you won't experience sore muscles. Jerry's response to this setup points out the humor in and futility of overexercising. He goes on to say something like: "So I have to train more so that exercise doesn't make me sore. Why don't I just stop exercising so that I never feel sore in the first place?"

Clearly Jerry didn't get addicted to exercise, but many do. Sometimes the things we love most are not necessarily good for us. When we jog, we may love it because it produces endorphins. If we jog too much and then feel sore the next day, we become addicted to jogging, because the endorphins produced take away the self-induced soreness. During jogging or any vigorous exercise, the more you hurt yourself, the more pleasure, power, strength, and exhilaration you feel.

> The more you hurt yourself, the more pleasure,
> power, strength, and exhilaration you feel.

Some young adults today go so far as to cut themselves or to pierce their bodies with hooks in their shoulders and then get raised up with a crane, suspended fifteen feet in the air. You would think that this is unbelievably painful, but they get high doing it. The pain quickly goes away because of all the endorphins the brain produces. Endorphins are natural painkillers.

Just as most Americans are horrified by this extreme behavior, the inhabitants of the mountainous areas of China, India, and South America, who commonly live well beyond a hundred years, view Americans in much the same light. They see us as obsessed with injuring ourselves by jogging and working out in gyms. From their perspective, we are unnecessarily shortening our life span.

Endorphins can be confusing. They are produced when we do good things for ourselves, but they are also produced when we are injured. When people get shot by a gun, they say it doesn't even hurt. When the body is *seriously* injured, the brain produces endorphins to take away the pain. People feel the pain the day *after* getting shot. Even though getting shot produces endorphins, it is still not a good idea to get shot every time you want to feel really good! In a similar manner, overexercising traumatizes the body to such an extent that the brain produces the intoxicating high that comes from endorphins.

Even though getting shot produces endorphins, it is still not a good idea to get shot every time you want to feel really good!

Endorphins are from heaven, because like angels, good parents, or teachers, they reward good behaviors but also comfort us when we have injured ourselves. Endorphins can be misleading. They are associated with winning, achievement, laughter, sex, love, happiness, enthusiasm, and excitement. They are the carrot that keeps us motivated to do good and be good.

EXERCISE, ENDORPHINS, AND A LONG LIFE

When we exercise, we produce endorphins. Endorphins are neurotransmitters produced in the brain that reduce pain and create feelings of happiness, vitality, and well-being. When endorphins are produced, we feel uplifted, fully alive, and inspired. We are high on life. We feel more connected with our purpose in life. We have a sense of being in tune with everyone and everything. The world is suddenly a much better place. In this sense, endorphins are from heaven.

We can easily become addicted to overexercising, because the brain produces extra endorphins to reduce the pain caused by stressing our muscles. The production of extra endorphins makes you high. The problem is that we have to injure ourselves to experience this ecstasy. Not only do we feel sore the next day, but we also put the body through unnecessary wear and tear. These actions shorten our life span and increase our chances of getting sick as we age.

Car engines are a good example of wear and tear. Generally speaking, a car engine has a predicted life span of a limited amount of miles. You could buy a fifteen-year-old car with only 10,000 miles, and it would be like buying a new car. Or you could buy a relatively new, overdriven rental car with more than 100,000 miles. This used rental car may look new on the outside, but its engine is going to wear out much sooner.

Overexercising may make you look like a newer model, but it puts a lot more miles on your engine. There are better ways to stay young, vibrant, and healthy. The body is designed to live for a hundred and twenty years. There are several societies in which people regularly live well beyond a hundred and are disease-free. The most well-known are the Hunza, who live in the mountains of Pakistan. These people do not live comfortable lives protected from stress. Each day they face the many stresses of survival under extreme weather conditions without all our modern conveniences. They live long, healthy lives, and they don't jog just for the exercise. Their longevity results from a healthful, mineral-rich diet, hard work, regular stretching, and long walks.

ENDORPHINS, STRESS, FOOD, AND EXERCISE

Endorphins are the body's first line of defense against physical, emotional, and mental stress. When you are faced with stress and your brain is well fed with nutrients, then your brain immediately produces extra endorphins to increase your sense of well-being. Stress on all levels—physical, emotional, and mental—will stimulate the increased production of endorphins. The stress from the outside world itself isn't the problem; instead, it is how our brain reacts to such stress. With healthy brain chemistry, stress stimulates well-being.

Endorphins are the body's first line of defense against physical, emotional, and mental stress.

When we exercise, we are choosing to stress our muscles. We are systematically *injuring* ourselves to stimulate the production of endorphins in our brain. This explains why exercise makes us feel so good. In moderation, this stress is good. Research has demonstrated time and time again that regular exercise decreases serotonin-deficiency symptoms of depression and anxiety, as well as such dopamine-deficiency symptoms as ADD and ADHD.

Regular exercise decreases symptoms of depression and anxiety.

One study demonstrated that a half hour of exercise three times a day is seven times more effective than prescription drugs in treating depression. Other research has demonstrated that thirty minutes of aerobic exercise along with vitamin supplements will remove the symptoms of ADD and ADHD in children. Prescription drugs may be necessary for some individuals. But for the millions of people who don't really need these drugs, regular exercise and nutritional supplementation are the solution.

A half hour of exercise three times a day is seven times more effective than prescription drugs in treating depression.

High concentrations of endorphins in the brain produce a sense of euphoria, enhance pleasure, and suppress emotional and physical pain. When endorphins are low, people may feel anxious. They are also more aware of pain. They crave sugar to produce relief by increasing serotonin, or they seek out fatty foods to produce endorphins. Endorphin deficiency in some is associated with an appetite for such fatty foods as french fries, cheese, creamy sauces, margarine, butter, fried chicken, potato chips, and chocolate, to name some of the most popular examples. After eating some fat, people notice a change in mood and feel more pleasure.

Moderate physical exercise, by burning stored body fat, raises endorphins and causes the same mood changes. By producing endorphins, exercise can also be an effective tool for controlling your appetite for the specific fats that are bad for you. By learning to eat plenty of *healthful* fats, you will stimulate endorphin production, burn fat, lose weight, and feel great. (We will explore good fats for your diet in Chapter 11.)

Emotional exercises can also produce endorphins. Millions of women every day receive the help of therapists to guide them through an exploration of feelings and emotions. As you remember feelings and process the pain of your past, endorphins are created and past issues get resolved. All of my books contain a variety of emotional exercises to stimulate the production of endorphins.

Emotional exercises can also produce endorphins.

THE FEELING LETTER

My favorite technique is called the feeling letter. Essentially the exercise is very simple. Whenever you are upset, if you want to feel better, simply write out what you are feeling.

On paper, write a letter to whoever is upsetting you. Within ten to twenty minutes, you will begin producing endorphins. Without editing yourself, write out your feelings associated with the four levels of negative emotion: anger, sadness, fear, and regret. Take at least two to three minutes to express anger, then sadness, then fear, and then regret. By taking a few minutes to exercise your ability to feel and express these natural healing emotions, you will feel immediate relief. To complete the process, exercise your ability to express positive feelings as well. Write out what you want, wish, love, appreciate, understand, and trust. You can file your letter or throw it away, but don't give it to the person with whom you were upset. Let it go and make up.

Twenty minutes of writing out your feelings will make almost anyone feel better.

In therapy or while journaling on your own, endorphins get produced as you remember and feel the pain of the past, and you begin to feel normal again.

Just as some people are addicted to exercise, others are addicted to emotional exercise or sharing painful feelings in therapy or with their friends. In moderation, physical and emotional exercise is good, but too much of anything is not a good thing. These addictive tendencies disappear when we find a healthier way to raise our endorphin levels.

ENDORPHINS AND MOTIVATION

Endorphins are your brain's way of rewarding you for using your body, feelings, and mind. If you challenge yourself and face life's stresses, you are rewarded by your brain. If you do not continue to grow in life, your brain doesn't reward you and does not produce endorphins. For most people as they age, mental, emotional, and physical pain increase. But if you continue to fully develop and use your many gifts throughout your long and healthy life, your brain will reward you with feelings of well-being caused by a consistent supply of endorphins.

Most people in the West are sufficiently motivated to do good things and be all that they can be, yet they still suffer from a variety of addictions. The real problem is not a lack of motivation but a nutritional deficiency. If you lack a healthy diet and exercise program, the pursuit of excellence in the ongoing process of developing your full potential is easily derailed by addictions, extreme materialism, and emotional poverty. People in the West have the education to know what is possible, but they don't have the nutritional support to make it happen and keep their lives and brains in balance.

The pursuit of excellence is easily derailed by addictions, extreme materialism, and emotional poverty.

Being motivated to live out our dreams stimulates the production of endorphins. We temporarily get high. We are inspired by a good teacher, role model, book, TV show, or movie, but it doesn't last. We taste the heavenly elixir of increased endorphin production, but if we don't get enough nutrition from our diet, our supply of endorphins runs out, and our endorphin high is followed by a crash.

In the West, we get higher, but we also crash lower. Since birth, we have been instilled with the healthy democratic belief that all men and women are created equal. We agree that we all have tremendous untapped potential and that we deserve equal opportunities to achieve success and happiness in life. We believe we are born with these basic rights of life, liberty, and the pursuit of happiness.

In the West, we get higher, but we also crash lower.

These messages ring the bell of truth within our hearts, and we are inspired to fulfill our mission in this world. In the West, we grow up in this context of ideals that can raise us up to the pinnacle of truth, justice, and integrity, along with the simple inspiration to be loving and good while making a difference in this world.

With this increased potential and the motivation to create heaven on earth, we also have the increased potential to live in hell. As I have explained, our lows are lower because our highs are higher. By flying so high, we deplete our supplies of endorphins and crash. Trying to fly up to the sun, we get our wings burned and come crashing down. To sustain a high level of endorphins, we must have enough raw materials. Without a nutritious diet, we don't have the fuel to make more endorphins.

When our supply of endorphins runs low, it takes more stimulation to create endorphins. Inspiring books and role models are not enough. The willingness to love and make a difference doesn't get us out of bed or help us to forgive and forget. Since our diet is not providing enough raw materials to fuel the production of more endorphins, many people live in a diet-induced hell.

Many people live in a diet-induced hell.

With a deficiency of endorphins, we live in a world of not enough time, energy, pleasure, and love. Natural endorphins restore a sense of abundance in life. The actual chemical makeup of endorphins is similar to the makeup of such addictive drugs as opium and morphine. Just as we become addicted to these drugs, we also become addicted to endorphin-stimulating behaviors.

When we are endorphin-deficient, any behavior that produces endorphins can become addictive. Any behavior done to the extreme will stimulate the production of endorphins. As a result, we become addicted to that behavior. The more endorphin-deficient we are, the more dependent we become on these extreme behaviors.

Since our food doesn't have the nutrition our body needs, we seek more food. We may go to work, but if that doesn't produce enough endorphins, we will resort to overworking. We may exercise, but if that doesn't produce enough endorphins, we will overexercise. To compensate for our deficit of endorphins, we will tend to *overdo* normal healthy behaviors.

ENDORPHINS AND STRESS

When the brain does not produce enough endorphins, the normal stresses of life become increasingly unbearable. Instead of bouncing back in response to stress with increased pleasure, confidence, and enthusiasm, we feel different degrees of physical pain, mental distress, or emotional despair. With endorphins, stress is our friend, but because of nutritionally deficient diets and lack of regular exercise, stress has become public enemy number one.

With low levels of endorphins, the normal stresses of life become increasingly unbearable.

This explains why endorphin deficiency prompts us to overdo normal healthy behaviors. Let's look at a few examples:

• By increasing physical stress to our muscles (exercise), we stimulate the production of more endorphins to reduce pain and restore well-being temporarily.

• By increasing mental stress by taking on too much work (deadlines and long hours), men in particular stimulate the production of endorphins to reduce mental distress and anxieties temporarily.

• By giving too much in relationships, women stimulate the production of endorphins to reduce emotional despair and depression temporarily.

• By eating more than the body needs, women in particular stimulate the production of endorphins to experience temporarily an island of peace in their day, generating feelings of comfort, contentment, and optimism. They are pushed to eat more by the serotonin-produced optimistic thought "I will have only one more cookie" or "I will go on a diet tomorrow."

Endorphin deficiency prompts us to excessive exercise, work, giving, and eating. The more deficient we are in endorphins, the more stimulation we need to feel good. If we are seriously deficient, we injure ourselves to produce the endorphins that will reduce our pain.

When overexercising allows us to experience immediate relief from the stresses of daily life, it is hard to stop. The more we overdo the behavior, the more we stimulate the production of endorphins. We don't realize that we have injured ourselves until the next day.

With a more balanced diet, we are not so dependent on extreme behaviors to cause injury. Instead, just moderate activity, work, giving, and eating are all enough to produce heavenly endorphins.

ENDORPHINS AND ADDICTIONS

For some people, exercise is addictive. This may sound harmless, but overexercising can be a serious addiction that disrupts our life, health, and relationships just as drinking, overworking, and overeating do. There is nothing wrong with regular exercise to stay fit, drinking in moderation to relax, working to make a living, and eating to sustain your body. These are all good things. They become a problem when we overdo them.

Excessive working and drinking on Mars and excessive giving and eating on Venus are the most common symptoms of low endorphin production. There are many more addictions, but let's focus on these four to get a sense of how men and women experience addictions differently.

Addictive tendencies are a symptom
of endorphin deficiency.

When men have low dopamine levels, longer hours and more challenging work will stimulate the energy, pleasure, and clarity of increasing dopamine. This then triggers the production of testosterone, which in turn triggers endorphins. The brain rewards increasing testosterone levels with more endorphins, which increase men's feeling of well-being. Who wants to stop feeling good, particularly if you have plenty of energy from increased dopamine? In this way, increased endorphins produce an addiction to work.

On Mars, the brain rewards increasing testosterone levels with more endorphins.

A similar circumstance occurs for some men when they drink alcohol. For some people, due to their unique genetic makeup, the body converts alcohol into dopamine. When this is the case, if you are already dopamine-deficient, one drink will cause your dopamine levels to rise and you will feel energized.

As dopamine levels rise, testosterone levels rise, and the brain rewards a man with increasing levels of endorphins. He suddenly feels more alive than ever before. He *has* to have more. Unfortunately, excessive alcohol consumption damages the liver and overstimulates the brain, producing many undesirable side effects.

When women have low serotonin levels, giving to others will stimulate the feelings of comfort, contentment, and optimism that come with increasing serotonin. This act of giving triggers the production of oxytocin, which in turn triggers endorphins in the brain.

On Venus, the brain rewards increasing oxytocin levels with more endorphins. These endorphins increase a woman's sense of well-being. Who wants to stop feeling good, particularly if you have plenty of love in your heart from increased serotonin? In this way, increased endorphins produce an addiction in women to giving too much.

On Venus, the brain rewards increasing oxytocin levels with more endorphins.

When women have low serotonin levels, eating more than their bodies need has the effect of raising serotonin levels. With a greater sense of calm, contentment, and optimism, a woman sustains a nurturing attitude toward herself. Through emotional eating, she comforts and nurtures herself with food. This nurturing behavior increases oxytocin levels, and the brain rewards this nurturing behavior by increasing endorphins. It feels so good that she just can't stop. In this way, she becomes addicted to endorphins as well as food.

Whether your brain is rewarding you for good behavior or protecting you from feeling the self-inflicted injuries of over-exercising, if your usual levels of endorphins are low, this sudden new surge becomes addictive. Whatever has stimulated the production of endorphins becomes your new drug.

ENDORPHINS, PROZAC, AND CORTISOL

Rather than using addictive behaviors or illegal substances to cope with the unbearable stress caused by low endorphin levels, millions of Americans ask their doctor for a prescription to take legal drugs. Taking prescribed drugs is just one step away from taking many common street drugs. LSD, PCP (phencyclidine), and other psychedelic drugs are serotonin-producing. PCP was a legal drug prescribed by doctors for seven years before it was banned by the government. It is now considered by the FDA to be one of the most dangerous drugs on the street.

Research shows that Prozac and similar serotonin-producing psychoactive drugs actually inhibit the pineal gland's ability to produce natural and healthy levels of serotonin on its own. So in addition to the long list of uncomfortable and dangerous side effects, prescription drugs actually disrupt your brain function.

Prescription drugs, just like alcohol and illegal drugs, have been shown to damage the liver. The liver is your body's biggest and most important organ. Its healthy functioning is essential in the processing of amino acids into healthy brain chemistry.

If that wasn't enough, there is more. Cortisol is a hormone produced by the adrenal gland in response to stress. It is called the stress hormone. Cortisol levels are naturally increased when we are under a lot of stress. High levels of cortisol give us extra focus and energy at times of emergency.

Everything from being behind schedule on a project, late for work, or stuck in traffic to recovering from a family argument, money worries, or a physically demanding job can cause an excessive release of cortisol. This results in accelerated muscle tissue breakdown and other negative effects throughout the body.

The production of endorphins not only relaxes us, makes us happy, and creates a sense of well-being, but also immediately lowers stress levels. This decrease of stress is measured in the body as decreased cortisol levels. Without endorphins to lower cortisol, our body lives in a state of perpetual hell.

A person taking serotonin-producing prescription drugs has increased levels of cortisol. They may think they are doing fine, but their bodies are totally stressed out all the time. This may help account for certain negative and undesirable side effects of such drugs.

A person taking serotonin-producing prescription drugs has increased levels of cortisol all the time.

High levels of cortisol are linked to elevated blood pressure, weight gain, an inability to build muscle, obesity, the development of diabetes, fatigue, depression, moodiness, and loss of sex drive.

High levels of cortisol are linked to high blood pressure, weight gain, and an inability to build muscle.

In the last ten years, obesity has become our nation's number-one killer. This epidemic of weight gain is also the basis of the historic and dramatic increase in diabetes during the last five years. Both these epidemics are associated with elevated levels of cortisol.

Long before anyone should consider long-term therapy for

depression or the more extreme measure of taking psychoactive drugs, he or she should get a personal trainer to help him or her exercise in a moderate manner. Regular exercise to produce endorphins and lower cortisol levels is far better than the possible damage that prescription drugs will do to your brain and body.

If you are taking drugs now, take heart. There are natural alternatives to help your body heal itself from the damaging effects of taking drugs. But stopping the use of prescription drugs can have more side effects than continuing to use the drug. You need to be under the supervision of a medical doctor who is informed about the possible side effects and will monitor your changing symptoms. In Chapter 13, I will explore this process of giving up drugs in greater detail.

Whether your symptoms are so severe that you depend on legal or illegal drugs, or if you depend on addictive behaviors, you can begin addressing this problem at its foundation. Rather than treat the symptoms, you can get to the cause. You already have built into your brain a perfectly designed hormone factory for reducing stress by producing endorphins. By making a few small but significant changes in your diet and exercise program, you can begin producing heavenly endorphins every day.

6

TESTOSTERONE AND OXYTOCIN: THE HORMONES OF WELL-BEING

Dopamine gives us clarity, energy, and motivation. Serotonin gives us comfort, contentment, and optimism. And endorphins increase our sense of well-being to help us to cope effectively with stress. These neurotransmitters are all directly determined by diet and exercise. Yet diet is not enough. There is more.

The quality of your relationships, communication, work, and lifestyle is also necessary for creating healthy brain chemistry. Effective and compassionate communication, a sense of cooperation from others, opportunities to work together with mutual support, and a spiritual community of like-minded people all stimulate the production of serotonin.

Opportunities to make a difference, positive feedback, acknowledgments, incentives, rewards, entertainment, friendly competition, challenging problems to solve, chances to innovate, and inspiring educational opportunities—all stimulate the production of dopamine.

The quality of our relationships and work directly stimulates the production of serotonin and dopamine from the raw materials provided by your diet. You may have the raw materials, but unless your relationships and lifestyle stimulate production, it doesn't happen.

The support we receive in relationships stimulates
brain chemicals from the raw materials provided
by our diet.

Receiving support in our relationships to increase our dopamine and serotonin levels is a requirement, but it is not enough to sustain well-being. To produce endorphins, we need also to give support. To achieve brain balance, we must balance giving and receiving, acting and achieving in our life. By giving of ourselves and doing our very best, we are able to stimulate the production of the hormones oxytocin and testosterone. In combination with healthy levels of dopamine and serotonin, this mixture creates heavenly endorphins.

No one can stimulate the hormones oxytocin and testosterone for us. This is a job we have to do for ourselves. To a great extent, we are dependent on others and externalities to stimulate the production of dopamine and serotonin. What we do and give in life determines our hormone levels. When a woman gives from a feeling of love, she is able to stimulate the production of oxytocin. When a man acts in the service of others to make a difference, he stimulates the production of testosterone. Increasing oxytocin helps to elevate and sustain serotonin levels; increasing testosterone helps to raise and sustain dopamine levels. By adjusting your behavior and/or your responses to a situation, you have the power to generate the right hormones to then stimulate the production of healthy brain chemistry.

RAISING HORMONE LEVELS

When hormones in the body rise to healthy levels, the brain rewards you with endorphins. Increasing testosterone is rewarded on Mars, and increasing oxytocin is rewarded on Venus. As we understand this unique biochemical difference in greater detail, we can understand why women and men behave and react in such different ways.

Endorphins are produced when
testosterone and oxytocin levels rise.

When a man acts in a way that is motivated to protect and serve, his levels of testosterone rise. To protect and serve, the Martian motto, is the motivation in every man's DNA. It is also the very behavior that stimulates testosterone.

Testosterone is the hormone of desire, and oxytocin is the hormone of love. Even when a man is not feeling very loving, if he remembers his desire to do the right thing and serves the well-being of others, his testosterone increases and his dopamine levels rise. When he gets positive feedback in response to his actions, his oxytocin levels rise as well, and he feels more loving.

This is not true for a woman. If she has low oxytocin levels and raises her testosterone levels by doing the right thing, she will have more energy from the increased dopamine, but she will not necessarily feel more loving. The problem for her is that increased testosterone and dopamine tend to lower her levels of serotonin and oxytocin. Instead of feeling better, she will feel even more deprived, hopeless, and unsupported.

A MAN'S SENSE OF WELL-BEING

If a man can do something to solve a problem, he immediately feels better. Doing something increases his testosterone levels. Increased testosterone releases endorphins in his brain, and as you know, more endorphins augment his well-being. For a woman, increasing testosterone by doing something can lead to lowering her oxytocin levels. Oxytocin levels generate the feelings of love and bonding. With less oxytocin, she is less able to appreciate the support she has and her motivation to care for others and share herself in love decreases. A dip in oxytocin leads to a decrease in serotonin, which will eventually reduce her feelings of well-being.

Whenever a man is doing something to achieve a
goal, he will feel better.

A man's well-being is directly tied in to his levels of testosterone. He becomes immediately energized when there is a problem to solve and he has the solution. When there is fire and he
has the water and hose, he is indeed a happy man. The fire
stimulates dopamine. Using the water and hose to put out the
fire stimulates testosterone. When a man has things to achieve
and accomplish, his testosterone levels rise and he is happiest.
When a man is feeling sexually aroused and he is confident that
he will achieve his goal, his increased energy and vitality add up
to increased happiness and pleasure. As the levels of testosterone
increase, endorphins in the brain are produced and the man's
sense of well-being increases.

BOYS FIGHT AND BECOME FRIENDS
AND GIRLS DON'T

Gender researchers have always found it curious that boys bond
after a fight or battle, but girls often become enemies for life.
The differences between the biochemistry of men and women
make these observations less mysterious.

When boys fight or demonstrate aggression, it is always to
protect someone or serve some cause. Whether a boy is protecting
or serving himself or others doesn't matter. His brain rewards this
increased testosterone with endorphins. Girls don't have the same
experience. There is nothing nurturing about a fight or battle.
Fighting is the opposite of communicating in a cooperative and
collaborative manner. For a girl, fighting results in more dopamine and testosterone, but her serotonin and oxytocin levels
drop. As a result, her sense of well-being is disrupted.

Two girls get into a fight, and because
serotonin and oxytocin levels drop, they become
enemies for life.

BALANCING WORK AND HOME FOR WOMEN

When men compete with each other with the intent to beat the other so that the best will win, it stimulates the good feelings of dopamine and increasing testosterone. Friendly competition is more clearly seen in sports, but it also rules the workplace to various degrees. Put a woman in a competitive work situation, and she doesn't derive the same hormonal benefits as a man. When her serotonin and oxytocin levels drop, her well-being decreases as well.

To balance the competition, aggression, risk, and challenge in the workplace, a woman is in greater need of a loving relationship when she gets home. She looks forward to sharing her feelings about the day, while her husband may want to forget his day and just enjoy some solitary activity like reading the newspaper, puttering in the garage, or watching TV. Sharing and communicating about his day is not a priority or a pressing need, because his serotonin levels are not abnormally low.

When she asks him about his day, he doesn't feel a need to talk or share; in fact he prefers not to. Particularly if he has had an exhausting day, he wants to take some time alone to relax and give his body a chance to restore his testosterone and dopamine levels. The last thing he wants to do is to talk about his day.

A woman looks forward to sharing her day, and a
man looks forward to forgetting his.

Some women may not want to share their feelings (particularly if their husbands talk a lot), but most do want to have a sharing and cooperative relationship. A woman wants to feel as though she can depend on a man's help and assistance in some manner.

All women are different in what stimulates their oxytocin levels, but oxytocin is the key to their feeling good. Likewise, testosterone is the key for a man. While most men don't want to talk about their day, some men do. Some men are very vocal when they get home from work. Talking helps them to restore testosterone levels. Talking about their day is an opportunity to make themselves right by complaining about someone or something that happened. Being right always increases testosterone levels.

Talking is a good thing for relationships, but too much talking by the woman or the man is . . . too much. Quite often, women married to these talkative men become less talkative and would prefer that their husbands talk less and help out more. If this is the case, he can still talk to his buddies. When he talks less, it will create the room for her to talk a little more, which is always good for her serotonin levels.

TESTOSTERONE, DOPAMINE, AND STRESS REDUCTION

In a boy or man, when testosterone levels go up, the brain rewards him with increased endorphins, and stress levels, as measured by cortisol, go down. Many men actually feel more relaxed and energized in the heat of the battle. Their biggest stress is waiting for the battle to begin.

Testosterone, the hormone of well-being for men, increases whenever they think they are protecting or serving. In reality, they may be committing a crime or even killing someone, but if they are convinced that they are ridding the world of a danger, their testosterone will increase along with their pride and sense of well-being.

If a man is convinced he is ridding the world of a danger, he will even enjoy killing and punishing others.

When testosterone levels go up and a man is not in the fighting mode to *protect* but in a supportive mode to *serve*, he is much more friendly, caring, and romantic. After a fight, a man can be ready for romance, but it may take days for a woman to recover and restore serotonin and oxytocin to healthy levels.

The relationship between testosterone and dopamine is reciprocal. Increased testosterone levels stimulate the production of dopamine, and increased dopamine levels stimulate the production of testosterone.

By initiating actions to serve a cause, a man experiences a release from the brain fog that commonly surrounds men with low levels of dopamine. High levels of dopamine are associated with clear thinking and focused behaviors. This increased dopamine then balances out his generally higher levels of serotonin.

By initiating actions to serve a cause, a man experiences a release from mental fog.

Dopamine focuses attention and serotonin expands the ability to take in and retain more information. Dopamine gives us the ability to prioritize and recognize what has to be done to achieve a goal or to execute a task. Dopamine stimulates the prefrontal cortex of the brain, which governs the rest of the brain. With normal dopamine levels, the executive part of the brain tells us what we have to do, achieve, and accomplish. In response, testosterone rises up and says, "Yes, sir. Let's do it now."

Testosterone is important to men because they are already so deficient in dopamine. Since women tend to have plenty of dopamine, testosterone is not as important. For women, stimulating oxytocin helps produce the serotonin they are deficient in.

When a woman is low in serotonin, she will overexpand, taking in too much information to stimulate its production. Too much information overloads her brain, limiting her ability to make sense of her situation or make decisions. Ironically, she feels an increased sense of uncertainty with more information. By performing oxytocin-stimulating nurturing behavior, she can relax as more serotonin gets produced. While nurturing, she is temporarily free from too much input in her brain.

Low serotonin causes us to overexpand,
taking in too much information to make
a decision.

When a man is low in dopamine, he will become overly focused on one thing—to stimulate production of dopamine. As he performs testosterone-producing behavior like solving a problem or lifting weights, his energy and pleasure levels increase as more dopamine is produced in the brain.

Dopamine focuses attention and
serotonin expands, taking in more information.

A dopamine-deficient boy who can't stay awake listening to his teacher will come alive playing a video game. This is because he is acting and getting reactions. This testosterone-producing activity stimulates more dopamine, and he suddenly has energy and focus.

A serotonin-deficient girl who is always trying to please others and cares too much about what everyone thinks will shift and become more relaxed when someone cares for her in a nurturing manner. Having a best friend is very important to a girl. Sharing secrets is a very intimate and oxytocin-producing behavior. When serotonin is low, the need for oxytocin is greater. Sharing secrets, when practiced to an extreme, can easily turn into cruel, cliquish behavior and negative gossip.

If you are hurt by someone, I can appear to be nurturing to you by agreeing with you and putting that other person down. When you are feeling mistreated, by criticizing the perpetrator and taking your side, I will begin to stimulate oxytocin in me and in you. In this way, girls with low serotonin compensate by forming cliques and excluding others.

For girls, having secrets is an intimate
and oxytocin-producing behavior.

With normal dopamine levels, we experience our intention to act to solve a problem, to achieve a particular goal, or to cause a particular outcome. Writing out goals or hearing someone talk about what is possible in the future stimulates the production of dopamine. We feel our call to action, and testosterone levels increase. Dopamine recognizes a solution to a problem and testosterone gives us the energy and motivation to solve it. With normal testosterone levels, we feel a sense of commitment, purpose, motivation, and energy.

KEEPING ROMANCE ALIVE

To keep the romance alive in a relationship, testosterone production needs to stay level as a man ages. Research shows that only in the Western world do men's testosterone levels drop as they age. In indigenous or rural communities around the world not exposed to Western food or farming practices, men's testosterone levels stay constant throughout life. They rise at puberty and stay up. It is probably the drop in dopamine that Western men experience that causes this drop in testosterone, which then causes the prostate troubles that men over fifty experience.

Men of the Hunza population in the mountains of Pakistan do not suffer prostate troubles, and they commonly produce offspring into their eighties and nineties. They are not even considered old or elders when they reach a hundred years.

**It is only in the Western world that
men's testosterone levels drop as they age.**

When a man leaves his high-stress job to return to his comfortable, loving relationship, his dopamine levels drop. Without sufficient dopamine levels, his testosterone levels begin to drop as well. If he gets the feeling that he is not doing anything or can't do anything to make his wife happy as he listens to her talk about her day, his testosterone levels drop even more.

When testosterone levels drop, an enzyme is released in a

man's brain that dissolves endorphins. When his endorphins are dissolved, his fatigue, inability to focus, and boredom turn into resistance. The more he tries to be empathetic, the more tired and bored he becomes. If and when he gives up trying, because he thinks that he can't make a difference, his testosterone levels drop dramatically and he becomes resistant, irritable, and angry. This anger and resistance signal that his endorphins have plummeted and his well-being has been disrupted.

When testosterone levels drop, an enzyme
is released in a man's brain that
dissolves endorphins.

To avoid sinking to this low level of well-being, a man is naturally motivated to stop listening and to seek some kind of dopamine stimulation long before he gets angry or frustrated. He can't wait to read the newspaper, watch TV, or do something. It is this urge to regain his well-being that motivates him to keep interrupting with solutions.

When he interrupts, it is not that he doesn't care. The truth is, the more he cares, the more depressed he becomes by passively listening and not doing anything productive to help. If he really didn't care, then not being able to help would not be frustrating at all.

The more a man cares, the more depressing it is
when a woman feels upset and he can't do
anything for her.

As men learn that women are from Venus and that they have different needs, much of this pattern can change. Instead of trying to solve her problems, he recognizes that what she needs most is simply to be heard. She is not looking for his solutions. He does not have to fix her or solve her problems. By listening, he *is* doing something.

Listening and not solving her problems is another
kind of doing: nonactive doing.

By listening and giving her an opportunity to talk, he helps her serotonin levels go up and her well-being increase. Instead of feeling passive, a man can easily be patient and recognize that he is making a difference. In this manner, his testosterone and dopamine levels go up instead of down. This simple insight makes a world of difference to stimulate the right productions of hormones and brain chemicals to sustain positive feelings in a relationship.

A man's serotonin levels rise when he gets home because he truly cares. This makes him content and satisfied but does not provide any challenge to stimulate dopamine. If his diet and exercise program doesn't provide him with an abundance of dopamine, his testosterone levels drop.

THE SIX STAGES OF DEPRESSION ON MARS

Statistically, women are three times more likely to become depressed than men are, and four times more likely to suffer seasonal depression. Ninety percent of the people who seek out counseling are women. These statistics make it seem as if women are much more vulnerable to depression. The truth is, men are just as prone to depression as women are. Men simply show their depression in a different way.

When he returns home, where there is not the intense stimulation of risk, danger, fighting, competition, and challenge, a man's energy level drops in a matter of a few minutes, and he feels fatigued. This low level of energy is actually the first stage of depression for men. This is similar to ADD or ADHD kids, who can't stay focused or energized while listening. In a classroom, they become tired, bored, and restless. These same changes occur when a man passively listens to his wife after a long day.

Let's explore the six major mood changes and the probable

biochemical causes associated with depression in a man. Keep in mind that these changes can be and are corrected with a diet and exercise program that can produce adequate levels of dopamine. We are speaking in general terms and these changes are not exactly the same for all men and boys. The six stages of depression are:

1. **Exhaustion and apathy.** Depression starts with not enough dopamine. With low dopamine levels at home or after work, a man will immediately feel tired. If his dopamine levels are normal, the little challenges of home life are enough to stimulate dopamine levels. But when his supplies of dopamine are depleted, a much bigger challenge or even an emergency is required to stimulate the normal levels of dopamine.

The more his wife complains, the more apathetic a man becomes. Even the thought of going home may make him tired. As soon as he walks in the door, he loses all motivation to do anything. He heads for a chair to sit and relax after a long day. From his perspective, his workday is over and he is just too tired.

2. **Inability to focus.** With his energy levels low, if he tries to be a good husband and connect with his wife and family, he will have difficulty focusing, listening, or remembering what to do. Trying to be helpful in some friendly manner increases his serotonin levels but lowers his testosterone levels. Brain scans reveal that when a man or boy with low dopamine attempts to focus, his prefrontal cortex suddenly becomes underactive. When he stops trying to focus, it becomes active again.

Without enough dopamine, a Martian has to try really hard to focus but can't. Although he can't focus, he does feel content and optimistic. He may even feel like laughing when he can't make sense of his partner's feelings. Serotonin makes us feel content, comforted, and optimistic.

3. **Boredom.** Testosterone is the urge to do it now. Serotonin makes us feel that there is no problem. As a man's serotonin levels increase, the urgency of testosterone dissipates and everything can wait till tomorrow. When serotonin increases, testos-

terone tends to decrease. Without the urgency to do something, a man begins to feel bored. With lower testosterone, he begins to feel restless, as if he should be doing something, but he doesn't know what. It is in this stage that men get caught in addictive habits.

4. Resistance. Lower testosterone signals enzymes in his brain to dissolve endorphins. A lower level of endorphins lessens his sense of well-being. This gives rise to feelings of impatience, annoyance, irritation, and anger. In relationships, this is when arguments heat up.

Women need to understand that even when a man is not depressed, his levels of testosterone are always fluctuating. We are all aware of a woman's monthly cycle, but most women and men are not aware that a man has a hormonal cycle that rises and falls every twenty minutes.

When a man is argumentative and grumpy, it is generally when his testosterone levels have dropped. Rather than argue with a man, an informed woman knows to back off for twenty minutes and then start again. At this point his levels will have risen and he will be much more cooperative, caring, friendly, and supportive. This twenty-minute cycle is normal for men, but may become less regular or more extreme with low dopamine levels. Knowing that a man's grumbles may dissipate in twenty minutes is very helpful for a woman. She mistakenly concludes that if he is annoyed, then he must be resentful. But annoyance in a man has little to do with resentment and can quickly pass.

5. Defiance. As his endorphins go down and his anger increases, his testosterone levels come back up as his serotonin levels drop. Without the sense of contentment and optimism provided by serotonin, he feels an urgency to do something. At this point he is not even angry. He is cold, uncaring, and aloof, not feeling anything. He is unresponsive to the needs and feelings of others as well as uncooperative. At this point, he is primarily defending and serving himself.

6. Meanness. As his testosterone levels increase, endorphins are produced in his brain, and as his serotonin levels decrease, his dopamine levels rise. His well-being increases as he focuses on disruptive, uncaring behavior; this can lead to meanness, cruelty, and criminal actions that are all justified in his mind.

This sixth stage is rare, but it explains why 90 percent of criminals in our society are men. It also explains the biochemistry of a serial killer. Research has revealed that serial killers have extremely low serotonin levels.

A quick review of these six common stages of depression follows:

Probable Biochemical Changes	Mood Changes
1. Dopamine levels drop.	**Exhaustion and apathy.** He feels tired and experiences low energy.
2. Dopamine levels are low and serotonin levels are rising.	**Inability to focus.** He tries to be a loving partner, but he can't focus. He may be forgetful and disoriented, but he does feel content and optimistic.
3. As serotonin levels increase, testosterone levels drop.	**Boredom.** With no focus or interest, he becomes bored and feels restless.
4. An enzyme is released in the brain to dissolve endorphins.	**Resistance.** He feels annoyed, irritated, and eventually angry.
5. Dopamine levels are still low, serotonin levels decrease, and testosterone levels increase.	**Defiance.** He does what he wants to do. He is unresponsive and uncooperative to authority and has little awareness of how his behavior will or does affect others.

Probable Biochemical Changes	Mood Changes
6. Dopamine levels rise, serotonin levels are low, testosterone levels are high, and endorphins are produced.	**Meanness.** His well-being increases as he clearly focuses on doing whatever he wants even if it is disruptive. This uncaring attitude can lead to meanness, cruelty, and criminal actions, which are all justified in his mind.

Most men live in the first two stages of depression when they come home. In the first stage, tired from the day, they don't even know that they are depressed. They think this state of low energy is normal. They have no idea that it has nothing to do with their day and everything to do with their diet and exercise program. Their low energy comes from a deficiency in dopamine.

In the second stage, faced with the prospect of coming home to a loving family, a romantic partner, a favorite TV show, or even to a loving dog, a man feels his serotonin levels go up. As a result of increased serotonin, he experiences real contentment, satisfaction, and an overall feeling of comfort. In this stage he is still depressed, but again he doesn't know it. He thinks it is normal to have no energy after a day at work, and he truly feels satisfied with himself and his life. Although his energy is depressed, he has no motivation to seek out help because he is feeling overall contentment in life. To him, there is no problem. Some call this the state of denial, while others consider it the bliss of ignorance.

Understanding the common symptoms of low dopamine and high serotonin in men at home gives new meaning to the old expression "Ignorance is bliss."

When he comes home, he is not focused and doesn't get much done. Without the stimulation of work, he doesn't really know what to do with himself. If he is married, he forgets to do the things he used to do. If he is single, he may conclude that he doesn't need more love in his life and will simply accept what is.

In the third stage of depression, he is bored and restless. This is not viewed as depression either, because it has a simple antidote. He can easily pacify himself by watching TV or reading the news or indulging in any other mindless behavior. He could also just drink a beer.

It is in this stage that addictions come into play. By keeping himself overstimulated, a man can avoid feeling bored and restless. A healthy addiction, like a hobby, can even help him to avoid moving on to the fourth stage of depression, but it is still not the best answer.

A healthy addiction, like a hobby, can even help a man avoid moving on to the fourth stage of depression, feeling angry.

With low dopamine, high serotonin, and low testosterone levels, instead of feeling motivated to participate in his family, a man feels satisfied, comfortable, and optimistic as he becomes a couch potato watching TV. When he sits down in front of the TV to relax after his long and hard day, he can relax and enjoy himself because his levels of serotonin are still normal, but he misses out on the ongoing pleasure of an active and enjoyable family life.

When asked to help out, he may feel put upon or at least resistant. Without enough dopamine, he doesn't have the energy to respond the way he would like. Certainly he wants to help, but he just doesn't have the energy. Often women cannot understand this. This is because women don't suffer from low dopamine unless they are depressed to the point of feeling unhappy, resentful, and very apathetic.

Sometimes a man does have the energy, but because he is not being asked to help, he just continues what he is doing. She is so used to him being in this low energy state that she doesn't even bother to ask. It can also be that she hasn't yet learned the importance of asking.

When a man doesn't help out, it is usually because he doesn't have the energy.

When women are depressed, their symptoms are complementary to a man's in the early stages. Just as men can't get up from the couch, women can't sit down and relax. He can't understand why she is so upset about things and overwhelmed, and she is bothered because he seems so uncaring, relaxed, and unmotivated. His response is relax, don't worry, and be happy. Her response is to take charge and do it all now. His thoughts regarding chores might well be "We can do it tomorrow," while she thinks it has to be done immediately or it will never get done.

Just as men can't get up from the couch, depressed women can't sit down and relax.

With low dopamine, a man finds his energy is limited. As a result, he doesn't do anything unless it *has* to be done from his perspective. This is not only frustrating to his wife but can make him feel worse as well. In the third stage, when he is feeling bored and restless, he needs to do something to stimulate testosterone; otherwise he will move into the fourth stage and feel angry and irritable. In the past, hobbies have helped men to overcome this challenge.

A man can just turn on the television and watch a football game. Research has shown that sitting and watching a football game or any engaging sport or action movie will increase a man's testosterone levels. This is just enough to pacify him and bring him back to stage two—low energy but happy.

If he doesn't move from stage three back to two, then he will inevitably move into stage four. This is when couples argue and fight and lose touch with their loving, kind, and compassionate feelings. If both partners do not recognize the need for a time-out, things start to get really ugly. He moves into stage five and argues in an uncaring manner. When this fails—and it will un-less they stop talking and he takes a time-out to restore his brain chemicals—he will eventually move into stage six and become mean. This is the stage at which domestic violence occurs.

THE SIX STAGES OF DEPRESSION ON VENUS

Women also go through different stages of depression as their hormones change. Let's explore the six major mood changes and probable biochemical causes associated with depression in women. Keep in mind that every woman is different and these are general patterns. The good news is that regardless of what chemical changes are happening in a woman's brain, balanced nutrition and exercise is the solution. This section is designed to help us understand the six stages of depression on Venus.

1. **Worry and discontent.** Depression starts with not enough serotonin. If serotonin levels are low and are not being stimulated, a woman will immediately begin to worry. If serotonin levels were normal, she could hold on to the optimism that she has plenty of support to deal with everything even when life is stressful. With depleted supplies of serotonin, she feels a much greater need to talk about all her concerns. When she doesn't get enough attention and empathy, her concerns increase.

2. **Feeling overwhelmed.** With increased worry and a feeling of not enough support, she feels an urgency to solve the problems associated with her concerns. Something has to be done, and it is up to her. This sense of urgency and increased responsibility stimulates her dopamine levels. With not enough time or support (low serotonin) and an increased sense of responsibility (increasing dopamine), she begins to feel overwhelmed.

Brain scans reveal that a woman feeling overwhelmed generally has an overactive brain. Serotonin relaxes and calms the brain. Without adequate levels of serotonin, her brain doesn't calm down. Normally, if serotonin reserves are not depleted, an overactive brain stimulates the production of more serotonin to relax the brain.

With increases in dopamine, instead of feeling relaxed, she feels motivated to do everything. Dopamine gives us energy and motivation, but when it is too high and serotonin is too low, the result is feeling overwhelmed by too much to do. She begins to feel helpless and hopeless.

3. Guilt and obligation. Oxytocin is stimulated when a woman feels free and relaxed to give in a nurturing manner. Dopamine creates the awareness of what has to be done immediately. Increasing dopamine and lower serotonin levels decrease her oxytocin levels. Without feeling supported by communication, cooperation, and collaboration, she feels she has to do it all herself, and her oxytocin levels drop.

As oxytocin levels begin to drop, she still feels she should be giving. She feels guilty for not giving more and then takes on more to do while neglecting her own needs. She is no longer giving freely, but instead gives of herself from obligation. In this stage, women will either overeat or give with strings attached, only to be disappointed again and again.

4. Resentment flu. Lower oxytocin signals enzymes in her brain to dissolve endorphins. Lower levels of endorphins lessen her sense of well-being. This gives rise to feelings of resentment. She may become critical, petty, or judgmental because she is doing it all and no one is helping.

At this point she gets resentment flu and is less willing to be so giving. She feels like a victim. Unless she is able to give and receive support, she will just spiral down into stage five.

This is the time when a woman needs to back off from expecting more from her relationship and give to herself. This is a time to stop blaming others for her unhappiness and take responsibility to make herself happy. This is also a good time to seek out the support of a therapist with whom to share her feelings, to talk or exercise with friends, spend time in nature, go shopping, dig into a good book, see a play, or go to a concert.

5. Exhaustion and apathy. She decides that it is not worth giving more because of her resentment flu. As a result of this decision, her levels of dopamine begin to drop. She is not willing to do it all. As her dopamine levels drop, she crashes into a state of exhaustion and apathy. She now feels less of an obligation to be good and giving.

At this point, no matter how supportive her partner is, she will just feel more resentment because she has given and now that he gives her a little, she is expected to be pleased. Her reaction to his apologies and offers to help is "Too late!"

6. Loss of self-respect. With decreasing dopamine, her serotonin and oxytocin levels begin to rise again. She figures that she is so tired that she is not going to be so responsible for others. At this point, she is somewhat liberated, with a new carefree feeling. Her new motto is "I don't care what others think."

With higher levels of oxytocin, her well-being increases but for the wrong reasons. She is happy because she doesn't feel obligated to give. The problem with this is that she stops feeling responsible altogether. She doesn't feel so dependent on others, so her serotonin levels begin to rise.

With low levels of dopamine and increasing serotonin, she loses her self-control and experiences increased impulsiveness. Most commonly she begins overeating and/or suffers from other eating disorders. She may turn on herself with disgust and self-hatred as she gives up her self-respect. With this low self-esteem, she may be attracted to or stay in abusive relationships. She cannot leave a destructive relationship, because she doesn't think she deserves better treatment. She may feel suicidal and in rare cases harm herself or others.

Let's review these common stages in a simple chart:

Probable Biochemical Changes	Mood Changes
1. Serotonin levels drop.	**Worry.** She feels worry and experiences not enough time, food, or support.
2. Serotonin levels are low and dopamine levels are rising.	**Feeling overwhelmed.** She feels an increasing responsibility to do it all. She feels pressured and overwhelmed.
3. As dopamine levels increase, oxytocin levels drop.	**Guilt and obligation.** She feels guilty not wanting to give more and gives more from obligation while neglecting her own needs.
4. An enzyme is released in the brain to dissolve endorphins.	**Resentment.** She feels critical, judgmental, or resentful because she is doing it all and no one is helping. She doesn't feel appreciated and gives less.
5. Serotonin levels are still low, dopamine levels decrease, and oxytocin levels increase.	**Exhaustion.** She now feels less of an obligation to be good and giving and crashes into a state of apathy and exhaustion.
6. Serotonin levels rise, dopamine levels are low, oxytocin levels are high, and endorphins are produced.	**Loss of self-respect.** This can lead to lack of control, overeating, self-abusive behavior, and/or staying in abusive relationships.

Most women live in the first two stages of depression. In the first stage a woman worries too much about herself and others. She is overly concerned about what other people think and is consistently discontented or anxious. She may be so used to this state that she doesn't even know what it is like to relax and have no worries. She mistakenly believes that she can't relax because she has so many things to worry about. She blames stress for her anxieties, not realizing that every person has the inner potential to relax as if nothing is wrong even when surrounded with problems. Problems cannot be avoided, but anxiety can.

Regardless of the stress in your life, you can relax as if everything will be okay.

In the second stage, she feels overwhelmed by too much to do and not enough time or support to get it done. She feels the urgency and motivation that comes with high dopamine, but lacks the optimism, contentment, and comfort that come with serotonin. This is the most common place for women to be. In this state, women are acutely aware of the problems in their lives, and they are motivated to do something about it. This is why so many more women seek out therapists than men.

Almost all women who are not medicated feel overwhelmed, with too much to do and not enough time.

Living in the second stage eventually leads to the third stage. With higher dopamine levels, her oxytocin levels begin to drop. Instead of freely giving of herself, she now begins to sacrifice herself and give from a sense of obligation or at least a hope that she will get more in return. This is a pattern that tends to happen in long-term marriages. She gives and gives until she gets to stage four and feels resentment flu.

When a woman notices that she is giving from obligation or she is starting to keep score, this is a warning sign that she is about to catch resentment flu. Turn around and start giving to yourself. If you keep giving with strings attached, you are setting yourself up to feel increasing resentment. This is the time for you to take a time-out from your relationship and focus on giving to yourself. Unless you turn around, it is all downhill toward increasing resentment, exhaustion, and loss of self-respect.

Feeling obligated is the warning sign to turn around; give more to yourself and not others for a while.

Depending on the degree of nutritional deficiency, these different stages can be more or less dramatic, and one could move very quickly or slowly through them. This insight will help you understand your moods and then gain control by giving yourself the support you need.

With the new and important insights of the Mars and Venus Solution, these later stages can be avoided. By applying *The Mars and Venus Diet and Exercise Solution,* both men and women can understand what happens in their relationships in a more positive light and can avoid all the stages of depression.

With this insight, changing moods, like natural weather patterns, are more predictable and start to make sense. You will be more motivated to make the changes in your diet and exercise routine. When it rains or storms, you will realize that it is not your partner's fault.

Instead of feeling powerless to create change, you will recognize that the power is in your hands. When the positive benefits occur, you will recognize them and understand why they are happening. This feedback is very important to keep you motivated to stay on the Mars and Venus Program every morning.

7

UNDERSTANDING OUR
DIFFERENT REACTIONS TO STRESS

In our culture, it has become common knowledge that our basic reaction to stress is the classic fight-or-flight response. When we encounter stress, a healthy person responds with increasing testosterone either to fight or to run away. The brain then rewards us for this activity with endorphins, and stress levels go down. This is true for men, but not as true for women.

Researchers are now beginning to realize that men and women have different coping mechanisms for dealing with stress. A recent landmark study at UCLA has found that women are far more likely than men to befriend in response to stress—that is to say, seeking social contact, with befriending methods ranging from talking on the phone or spending time with relatives and friends to such simple exchanges as asking for directions when lost.

Women ask for directions when lost as a way of raising oxytocin levels and reducing stress.

In particular, the research team points to the hormone oxytocin as playing a large role in the tend-and-befriend response. In the past, oxytocin has been studied largely for its role in childbirth, but it is secreted by both men and women as a response to stress. The calming effects of oxytocin in men are reduced by increasing testosterone levels.

This recent research reveals that oxytocin plays a key role in reducing a woman's response to stress by buffering the fight-or-flight response and encouraging her to tend to her children and gather with other women instead. Studies suggest that more oxytocin is released when a woman actually engages in this tending and befriending, which produces a calming effect.

TO CARE AND SHARE

Certainly a woman can and will fight to defend herself. Fighting may keep her safe and alive, but it doesn't necessarily lower her stress levels. However, all the caring, nurturing, and sharing after the battle will lower her stress levels. Caring and sharing behaviors increase the hormone oxytocin.

By caring and sharing in friendship, a woman produces oxytocin and stress levels go down.

This research confirms the link between oxytocin and stress for women and not for men. The researchers coined the phrase the *tend-and-befriend response* to describe a woman's response to stress. By tending to others—caring, sharing, listening, helping, nurturing, teaching, guiding, healing, feeding, grooming, cleaning—a woman experiences a rise in oxytocin levels, and her stress diminishes.

By befriending others, a woman also stimulates oxytocin. Making peace is a woman's first reaction to stress. Having to protect, defend, and fight causes a woman's stress levels to go up. If there is danger, her reaction is "Let's try to work things out." As she acknowledges her intent to bond and connect, a woman's stress levels go down. This occurs by means of communication, cooperation, and collaboration.

> As she communicates, cooperates, and
> collaborates, a woman's oxytocin levels increase.

This research explains why women tend to give more when stress levels go up. Women seek to give to and nurture others or they form friendships to share, cooperate, and collaborate. This sense of community gives women a feeling of safety and support, causing oxytocin levels to rise.

TO PROTECT AND SERVE

When a woman's brain hormones are in balance, a confrontation is certainly not a woman's first choice in dealing with stress. Fighting is not necessarily the first choice for a man, either. Fight or flight is actually one of the many ways a man will seek to protect and serve. From a more enlightened perspective, protect and serve is a man's reaction to stress, and not fight or flight. Fight or flight is what a man does at last resort.

> Fight or flight is one of the many ways a man will
> seek to protect and serve.

A woman's reaction to stress is to care and share. Her last resort is often the opposite of fight or flight: it is to fake or fold. Women are masters of makeup and disguise. They are so good at masking their own feelings from others that they often fool themselves. In the name of creating harmony and positive feeling, women will often pretend to be more loving and cooperative than they want to be.

> Fake or fold is one of the many ways a woman
> will seek to care and share.

Women are also masters of sacrifice, or giving in for the sake of harmony. Men can and will make sacrifices, but they will do so only when there is some definite reward, achievement, or purpose. Men pick their battles and sacrifices depending on what is most important. Women will sacrifice without even being aware of it. The number one pattern a woman has in her relationships when problems arise originates from giving too much and then resenting later that she didn't get back what she felt she deserved.

Women give too much and then later feel resentful.

Fake or fold is only a woman's last resort. A woman's primary stress reaction is her response to care and share. To acknowledge and deepen her bond with another, she will freely give what she herself would appreciate most. To sustain this caring and giving attitude, she needs to get back. This sharing creates an oxytocin-producing bond.

Women most easily bond with young children because they recognize the helplessness of a child and don't expect anything in return. Their supply of oxytocin becomes more limited as their expectations and requirements for receiving support back increase. As a woman's serotonin levels rise to normal through a healthy diet and exercise routine in the morning, she has a greater awareness of the support available in her life and doesn't expect so much in return from her romantic partner.

OXYTOCIN, SELF-NURTURING, STRESS, AND LOVE

The oxytocin response also occurs when a woman does something nurturing for herself. This is one of the most important lessons for a woman. It is easy to love and care for others, but not so easy to love and care for herself. So often women give and give but don't take time for themselves. Giving to yourself is just as important as giving and being there for others. Have you ever had a good cry and felt great afterwards? By feeling compassion for yourself, you felt better. You felt better because oxytocin levels increased and endorphins were produced to reward you.

Shopping in an unhurried manner is another example of an oxytocin-producing treat for women. Any behavior that a woman doesn't *have* to do but loves to do is an oxytocin self-nurturing behavior. If she feels she has to do the same behavior, it is dopamine-producing and serotonin-decreasing. When she acts from obligation, it encourages the belief that she doesn't have enough time and support in her life.

**Any behavior that a woman doesn't *have*
to do but loves to do is an oxytocin
self-nurturing behavior.**

Women lessen their stress levels by reaching out to bond in relationships through communication, cooperation, and collaboration. A woman's greatest source of stress is a loss of bonding or low oxytocin levels. Without love, a woman is not happy.

**A woman's greatest source of stress
is a loss of bonding or low oxytocin levels.**

Love in this context is the affirmation of the bond, the active acknowledgment of having a bond. Love is fully embracing our connection with someone or something. When we love someone, we acknowledge that that person is special to us. We seek to give him what we would want. Through caring, nurturing, and sharing with another, a woman reinforces her bond by giving exactly what she would want.

Self-nurturing and self-love also stimulate oxytocin. It is important to love others, but it is even more important for a woman to love herself. By taking the time to nurture herself along with her relationships, she is ensuring that she doesn't end up feeling used and abused.

Giving without getting back is actually one of our greatest joys and freedoms in the world. This can be realized only when we are fully capable of loving ourselves. Each time a woman chooses to nurture herself rather than indulge in resenting others, she is not only creating the immediate relief that comes from self-nurturing, but she is maturing in her ability to love herself. Ultimately this self-love frees her to give love all the time.

Giving without getting back can be one of
our greatest joys and freedoms in the world.

By taking time every morning for her self-nurturing diet and exercise routine, she will be building this solid foundation. Not only will she be getting the nutrients and stimulation necessary for the production of healthy brain chemistry and hormones, but oxytocin will be stimulated because she is taking the time she needs for herself. This is the best use of her time. By giving herself ten to thirty minutes of exercise and making sure to supply her body with nutrients at breakfast, she will be much more capable of giving freely of herself throughout the day.

LOVING A MAN FROM MARS

When a woman loves a man, she makes the mistake of giving him what she would want. Men certainly enjoy some caring, nurturing, and sharing, but what they want most are different expressions of love. Being testosterone-based, a man needs expressions of love that stimulate his testosterone and dopamine levels. These expressions of love are also present in a woman's heart when she loves a man, but she doesn't realize how important they are to him. They are the feelings of appreciation, acceptance, and trust.

A man needs expressions of love that stimulate his
testosterone and dopamine levels.

These three loving feelings promote the production of testosterone in a man. They are the emotional expressions that acknowledge to him that he is, can be, or will be successful in protecting and serving her. They acknowledge that with his support, she has, can have, and will have her heart's desire. This feedback feeds the fire of a man's desire to serve and protect. As his testosterone levels go up, his stress levels go down.

Appreciation, acceptance, and trust promote the production of testosterone in a man.

Serotonin allows the brain to recognize what it has, can have, and will have. Normal serotonin levels are associated with contentment, comfort, and optimism. These are all states of having. Most depression has to do with the feeling "I don't have, I can't have, or I will not have." The positive sense of having is necessary to feel the acceptance, appreciation, and trust that will support her partner the most. It is not only the symptom of feeling safe, loved, and supported, but it is also the symptom of increasing serotonin levels.

Depression has to do with the feelings "I don't have, I can't have, or I will not have."

When serotonin levels are normal, we are content with what we have, comforted by what we can have, and optimistic about what we will have. These same three recognitions associated with serotonin give rise to exactly the kind of love that men want and need most. These three states of havingness give rise to love in the following ways:

• Contentment with what you *do* have gives rise to the feeling of appreciation. When a woman is appreciative of what she has, it inspires a man to give more.

• Comfort with what you *can* have gives rise to the feeling of acceptance. When a woman is accepting of what a man provides (and doesn't seek to change him or correct him), a man gets megadoses of what he needs most. Her acceptance motivates him to learn from his mistakes and give more.

• Optimism about what you *will* have gives rise to the feeling of trust. When a woman trusts a man's intentions and believes that he can deliver, he gets the emotional support he needs most.

Men are always taking credit for things because they have such a great need to feel trusted as someone you can depend and rely on. A woman with low serotonin levels finds it hard to give this trust. Instead, she worries too much, giving him the message that he is not trusted or that she expects too much. No man is perfect, nor should he be expected to be.

Men are always taking credit for things because they have such a great need to feel trusted.

Often a woman thinks she is trusting a man by not asking for what she wants. When she wants more, she will not ask for it, and then feels disappointed when he didn't give it to her. She secretly feels that if he really loved her, he would do what she wants without her having to ask. This would probably happen if he was also from Venus, but he is from Mars and he doesn't think the way she does. He doesn't know what she wants.

The true expression of his caring is not that he anticipates her needs, but that he does his best when she does ask for his support. Certainly it is great when he offers his support without her having to ask, but if he doesn't, she should remember it doesn't mean he doesn't love her or care.

When he doesn't offer the support she is looking for, a way for her to nurture herself and give him the support he wants is for her to ask. Asking actually expresses a trusting attitude. She trusts that she will get help if he can give it. By not feeling hurt or upset if he can't give it, she is trusting that he would if he could. When she asks for support, it affirms her belief that he is willing and available to protect and serve her in some manner.

Asking for support can express a woman's trusting attitude.

If her need for help seems obvious, but he is not offering his help, he probably doesn't know it is required. Just the other day, Bonnie and I were leaving our ranch. Bonnie was carrying a bunch of last-minute items in her arms she had picked up on her way out to the car. I was carrying nothing and didn't even think about offering to carry these items. Two other Martian friends were with us, and they didn't offer either. It was not that we weren't willing. We just didn't think of it. We were busy talking about something. When she asked for help, everyone was happy to give it. This is a little issue, but it is very important.

From the Mars side, whenever you can be of assistance to a woman, offer it. From the Venusian side, if you would like assistance, ask for it. Even if you *can* do it by yourself, by asking for and getting support, you will be bonding; oxytocin and serotonin levels will go up. When a woman gives a man the opportunity to help in little ways, the appreciation she feels will stimulate good feelings in him as well.

Being asked for help stimulates testosterone in a man, and being offered help stimulates oxytocin in a woman.

In a variety of ways, women think they are being supportive to a man. They give what they would want, but it is not the kind of love a man wants. A woman gives oxytocin-producing love but omits the testosterone-producing love. These are a few examples:

- She may express worry and concern as a way of saying she cares, but he hears that she is not trusting him.
- She may ask a lot of questions to increase their connection and demonstrate her caring and understanding, but he hears she doesn't trust him and probably wants to help him in some way.
- She will offer her assistance at times when he is not asking for help, and he gets the message that he is not trusted to do something on his own.

A woman looks for opportunities to help a man to demonstrate that she cares for him. When she wants to help and he has not asked for help, he may easily get the message that she doesn't accept or appreciate his way of doing things. Her attempts to help are sometimes interpreted as her trying to teach him or correct him.

On her planet this is love, but it is not love on his. With the education provided in my different Mars and Venus books, a woman can learn to demonstrate her love in a manner that is more appropriate on Mars. Not only will he get more of what he wants, but this exercise will also increase serotonin production in her brain.

Testosterone is the hormone of desire. It is the active acknowledgment of what has to be done. While love acknowledges what we have, desire acknowledges what we have to do, achieve, or accomplish. When a man gets the feedback from a woman that his attempts to love her are appreciated, accepted, and trusted, then he feels a greater desire to be more, do more, and have more. Women inspire men to desire more.

Women inspire men to be, do, and have more.

The secret in loving a man is to ignore his mistakes and shortcomings whenever possible and respond instead to his successes. A woman should not try to accept, appreciate, or trust a man's weaknesses and limitations. That would not be honest. Instead, she should minimize their importance by focusing on what she does appreciate, accept, and trust. A trusting, accepting, and appreciative attitude makes a woman attractive to a man. It brings out the best in him and helps him to see and cherish the best in her.

MEN ARE LIKE RUBBER BANDS

Men also benefit from oxytocin, but too much is not as good for men. Too much oxytocin will reduce his testosterone levels.

When his testosterone levels are reduced, his levels of desire, motivation, and energy drop. This is most dramatically seen in physical intimacy. At the time of climax, both the man and woman experience a moment of bonding that dramatically increases oxytocin. This is certainly a rejuvenating experience for men and women. The difference is that the bonding will lower a man's testosterone and dopamine levels so much that when he is done, he falls right to sleep.

The woman, however, is fully energized and would like to continue cuddling and being close. Her body floods with oxytocin, and she benefits from lowered testosterone and dopamine levels. Remember, women become overwhelmed when their dopamine levels are higher than their serotonin levels. Dopamine tells us we have to do something and testosterone says it needs to be done now. With lower Martian hormones, she can relax and enjoy her need to love and bond.

After climax, a woman floods with oxytocin and fulfillment, and a man falls asleep.

Unless a man has strong testosterone and dopamine levels, with increased levels of oxytocin, his testosterone drops and he suddenly feels the symptoms of low dopamine syndrome. At the very least, he will feel his need for more space to recover and replenish his dopamine and testosterone levels.

This explains the rubber band theory I explore in my book *Men Are from Mars, Women Are from Venus.* After men get close, they then feel the need to pull away. When they stretch away like a rubber band, they will feel a strong desire to get close again after some time.

After men get close, they then feel the need to pull away.

When a man pulls back, he is seeking his space and a sense of autonomy in his life. This breathing room stimulates the production of testosterone and dopamine. Whenever a man is on his own and has to do things by himself, his testosterone and dopamine levels increase and his oxytocin levels decrease. When testosterone levels are high, he will once again have the energy, desire, and confidence to protect and serve. He wants to be in a relationship to give freely of himself by protecting and serving.

As a man gives more and gets closer and closer, his oxytocin levels go up and gradually his testosterone levels go down. At this point he needs to pull away, get some space, and then come back. With this insight, women don't have to take it personally when a man pulls back. When he says it is not her, he is telling her the truth. It is simply his need to balance his hormones again.

LOVING A WOMAN FROM VENUS

When a woman responds in a way that is motivated to care and share, her oxytocin levels go up. To care and share is the Venusian motto. This is why women commonly overgive. When women are stressed, instead of relaxing and giving less, they feel a compulsion to give more. This giving more creates increased oxytocin in her body, which then stimulates endorphins, which then lessens her stress. When love is a one-way street for her, it is not sharing. If she feels that she is not getting back what she is giving, her oxytocin levels drop. Keeping those levels of oxytocin up is the secret to loving a woman from Venus.

Instead of relaxing and giving less when stressed, women often feel a compulsion to give more.

When a man learns how to reciprocate, to give back the love she gives to him, he will hold the secret to keeping her happy. Too much emphasis in the world of psychology is put on men becoming more sensitive and opening up in relationships. Of course men are going to resist these behaviors. To support their partners more effectively, men don't have to become like women.

A woman doesn't need her man to be her girlfriend. Even if she thinks that is what she wants, it is not healthy, and it would eventually put out the fires of passion. Differences attract us to each other, and respecting and appreciating our differences sustains this attraction.

A woman doesn't need her man to be her girlfriend.

By understanding the little things that have a big effect on women, a man can make the difference in a relationship without trying to change his basic nature. Likewise, by learning how to respond to a man's actions, a woman can get what she needs without needing to change his basic nature.

A man's masculine traits actually help to balance a woman's hormones. Anytime a man uses his testosterone to protect and serve the woman he loves, he stimulates in her *both* oxytocin and testosterone. This is the balanced response that can emerge in a loving and supportive relationship. When we achieve a balance of testosterone and oxytocin, our sense of fulfillment is maximized. Balance always brings out the best in us. This understanding of a woman's different hormones and interests helps a man to achieve this end.

A woman's well-being is tied to her levels of oxytocin in a variety of ways. You can see a woman's face light up when she interacts with a baby or child. She doesn't mind giving without expecting back from a baby, because she knows the baby cannot give back to her. It is completely vulnerable and dependent. The glow on her face is rising oxytocin levels. This same glow occurs when she eats chocolate, receives a compliment, or gets a hug or massage. What do all these activities have in common? They all stimulate higher levels of oxytocin in her body. Chocolate actually produces serotonin, but as her serotonin levels increase, so do her oxytocin levels. Giving hugs and getting a massage directly stimulate oxytocin production by stimulating a woman's skin and the layer of fat just beneath the skin surface. This stimulation is generated through a massage or an affectionate but nonsexual touch. A woman needs to be touched several times a day.

Giving hugs and getting a massage directly stimulate oxytocin production.

Receiving compliments increases her levels of serotonin, which in turn increases her oxytocin levels. When someone is nurturing or friendly to a woman, she feels motivated to nurture in return. When she receives small gestures of affection, she feels safe to care and share in return. The anticipation that she will get back warm and friendly support makes it safe for her to nurture and share. Increasing oxytocin releases in her brain the endorphins of well-being that help to minimize the effects of stress.

Oxytocin is important to men but not nearly as important as it is to women. Here are a few examples of oxytocin-stimulating behaviors that men generally don't engage in:

- Men generally don't light up when they see babies, nor do they talk about wedding showers. The cells in their bodies don't long to cradle a baby in their arms.
- Men generally don't hug after business meetings, but they will make jokes and congratulate each other.
- Men generally don't give compliments on a basketball court about each other's outfits. A man generally doesn't notice or care if his teammate has new shorts to match his new shoes.
- Men generally don't notice when a friend gets his hair cut. Not only do women notice, but they may feel a little hurt if you don't notice.
- Men generally don't rejoice in having to shop for presents well in advance, wrap them, and buy cards. Most men would rejoice if Valentine's Day didn't happen every year.
- Men like massages, but they don't frequent spas the way women do, nor do they pamper themselves with regular facials or pedicure treatments.

- Men generally don't talk about wedding plans and fuss over all the details.
- Men generally don't volunteer to make cookies for the school bake sale.
- Men generally don't feel hurt if an old friend doesn't call for ten years and then happens to call.
- Men generally don't offer to carry something for a friend unless he asks.

The list of oxytocin-stimulating behaviors goes on and on. Since oxytocin tends to lower testosterone levels, such behaviors are just not so important to a man. When he doesn't seem to be as nurturing or sharing as a woman, it is not that he doesn't care about her, it is because different types of stimulation help him to cope with stress.

What is more energizing for him is solving problems, making money, achieving success, taking risks, facing danger, taking credit, being right, having the right answer, knowing the way, doing things on his own, having a special skill or department, making decisions for himself, being efficient, getting to the bottom line, acting to save others, making a difference, viewing action movies or sports, keeping score, enjoying competition, or looking at erotic pictures of the opposite sex. What do all these activities have in common?

These are all testosterone-producing behaviors. Women certainly engage in them, but for women they are often stress-causing situations. They may cause stress because they lower her oxytocin. For men, these activities are generally stress reducers if their dopamine levels are normal. Any behavior that raises testosterone in a man will give him energy and produce stress-reducing endorphins in the brain.

BALANCING HORMONES

It takes a deliberate intention for one behavior to sustain both oxytocin and testosterone levels. Lovemaking is the best example of balancing these complementary hormones. If a man follows his basic instincts, which are governed by testosterone, the whole process may take only five minutes. A man balances his hormones by taking more time for foreplay in the bedroom, twenty to thirty minutes instead of three to five minutes. By deliberately slowing down to respect a woman's different needs, he is being considerate (oxytocin) and he is staying focused on his goal (testosterone).

In the work world, balancing hormones in one behavior is much more challenging. Here are some examples:

- It is difficult to be cooperative (oxytocin behavior) while you are also being competitive (testosterone behavior).
- It is hard to be collaborative (oxytocin behavior) when you have to do something all by yourself (testosterone behavior).
- It is nearly impossible to listen to someone and his or her feelings (oxytocin behavior) when you are facing a deadline and you need to find a solution right away (testosterone behavior).

In spite of these challenges, the more balance we can bring into the different areas of our lives, the healthier and happier we will be. I address this challenge in much greater detail in my book *Mars and Venus in the Workplace*. We have an easier opportunity to find this balance in a relationship. We can't always choose the people with whom we work, but we *can* choose the people with whom we spend our personal life.

Balance is essential because testosterone and oxytocin are complementary. Their relationship is like a seesaw. When one goes up, the other goes down. With normal levels of serotonin, a woman finds it much easier to sustain both hormones at the same time. If she feels comforted, contented, and optimistic (increased serotonin), then testosterone-producing behaviors on her part do not negate her more nurturing oxytocin-oriented feelings and responses.

**Testosterone and oxytocin are complementary:
when one goes up, the other goes down.**

Likewise for a man. With normal levels of dopamine, oxytocin-producing behaviors don't negate his testosterone-stimulating behaviors. He is capable of being patient and considerate, yet getting to the point. He can freely give of himself and also think about what he wants for his reward.

It is interesting to note that when a man has sex with a woman he deeply loves (high serotonin and oxytocin), he will tend to have a greater drop in testosterone afterwards and for the next few days. If he really doesn't care that much for her, his testosterone may not drop as much. If he does not care at all, it may even go up.

This is evident in the lives of athletes. Sex with someone they love clearly lessens their aggression the next day. For this reason, coaches ask a man to abstain from sex the night before a game. Unmarried and rather promiscuous athletes report that sex the night before can stimulate even more testosterone and aggression the next day. It all depends on how close a man feels to his partner. Biochemically speaking, it depends on how high his oxytocin and serotonin levels get. When oxytocin is low, dopamine and testosterone can stay high.

**Unmarried and rather promiscuous athletes report
that sex the night before a game can stimulate
even more testosterone.**

The challenge in our relationships is to achieve a balance of these neurotransmitters so that hormone levels do not drop. To achieve this balance, men and women are greatly assisted by a dopamine-producing diet for men and a serotonin-producing diet for women. Learning to give and get the necessary emotional support to stimulate and balance the production of dopamine and serotonin is essential as well.

I used to hold three-day and seven-day seminars to create a safe and nurturing environment for men and women to process unresolved feelings from their past. In these seminars, after all the tears, people would be teleported to a heavenly state. The result of all their explorations and sharing was increasing oxytocin and endorphins.

In these seminars, men enjoyed the endorphin high just as much as women did. A man's brain also rewards him for increased oxytocin. The problem for a man is that if his testosterone levels are not also strengthened, he will lose this high feeling. Increasing oxytocin tends to lower a man's testosterone levels. If he doesn't have a lot of stimulation in his life to produce testosterone, his levels will drop and enzymes released in his brain will dissolve his endorphins.

If he has low dopamine levels, as most men do, he is even more vulnerable to the loss of testosterone after being nurturing to others. The emotional high of increased oxytocin is followed by a low. In my seminars, I learned that to help men sustain this high, I had to balance oxytocin-producing exercises with testosterone-producing exercises.

Increasing oxytocin tends to lessen testosterone,
and lower testosterone decreases a man's
well-being.

This same pattern is true for women in the reverse. A woman may enjoy the endorphin high from being very testosterone-oriented in her work responsibilities or from a rigorous exercise routine, but without a balance of oxytocin activities she will lose her high. Whether she is working on a construction site or at home raising little children, being responsible for the well-being of others stimulates a lot of testosterone and lessens oxytocin, particularly when she is in charge or if she doesn't have much help. Autonomy or doing things on your own stimulates dopamine and testosterone but lessens oxytocin. This increased testosterone is rewarded by the brain, but it also lowers oxytocin.

If a woman doesn't have enough activities to stimulate oxytocin, then the well-being from increasing testosterone doesn't last. Finding balance for both men and women is an important challenge if we want to stay stress-free and healthy.

Increasing testosterone tends to lessen oxytocin, and lower oxytocin decreases a woman's well-being.

When it comes to balancing hormones, the big difference between men and women is that when men have low oxytocin levels, their brains don't reduce their endorphins. If a woman has low testosterone levels, her brain doesn't take away her endorphins. Low testosterone is a major source and cause of stress in men, and lower levels of oxytocin are a major source of stress for women. This distinction makes men more work-oriented and women more relationship-oriented.

This distinction has not yet been explored by modern researchers, but once you learn to recognize the mental and emotional symptoms of the different hormones and neurotransmitters, it becomes obvious.

My favorite example to point out how endorphins are reduced when testosterone levels drop in a man but not in a woman comes from my experience at the movies.

DRIVING TO *THE BRIDGES OF MADISON COUNTY*

One Sunday afternoon, I took my wife, Bonnie, to see the movie *The Bridges of Madison County*. This was definitely a chick flick. As an expert on gender differences, I thought that since this was a book that millions of women had read, I should at least see the movie. I also knew it would put my wife in a great mood. The theater was packed with women; two other men were also there. There wasn't an empty seat. A few minutes after the movie started, there was a bustling noise of purses opening as the women searched for tissues. Some were already starting to cry in anticipation of the moments when they would cry again. For the women in this theater, this movie was a love fest.

I was also set for a good experience. After all, Clint Eastwood was the lead Martian. He is a reliable action figure. He wouldn't let us fellow Martians down. Five minutes after the movie started, I began to get tired, and I wasn't tired before I went in. Just watching this movie, with no action and all talking, was wearing me out. My eyelids were getting heavier and heavier. I couldn't believe it. I looked around, and all the women were completely attentive and alert. They looked like men watching an action film.

**Just watching a movie with no action
and all talking can wear a man out.**

For these women, there was a lot going on. They were already wondering what he was going to say, how she was going to respond, what she was thinking, what he was thinking, what was her husband going to think, how she felt about her husband, would she leave her husband, would Clint stay for her, was he finally going to settle down, what her fears were, was he afraid of intimacy, could she heal his broken heart, what was her life like up to that moment, what would her life be like if he left, what would happen to her marriage if they kissed, did he want to kiss her, would he make the first move, would she make the first move? Such suspense, such excitement, such a buildup. I looked over at the two other men, and they too were falling asleep.

For the women, a lot was going on, but for the men, nothing was happening. At a later point, as I struggled to stay awake, I suddenly got a second wind. It was as if I had just eaten some ice cream or drank a cup of coffee. My energy was back. What had happened? Well, something finally happened in the movie. Clint got in his truck and drove to the bridges. But when nothing happened there, my fatigue was back.

After I shared this story at one of my seminars, a man came up to me. He told me that he too had had the same experience but had more to add. He said, "I also got my energy back when Clint got in his truck, but then when he finally got to the bridge, he didn't even blow it up."

We laughed, and I completely agreed.

At the end of the movie, Clint Eastwood got in his truck to drive off into the sunset. I suddenly awoke from my slumber. As I looked around, more tissues were being passed out, and my wife's face was glowing with oxytocin. Once I had the opportunity to leave the theater and get in my car, my testosterone levels would recover. With the glow on her face and the increasing testosterone levels back in my body, we had a *very* nice evening.

Sleeping through *The Bridges of Madison County* is a great example of how a man loses his vitality and a woman doesn't when oxytocin and serotonin levels rise and testosterone levels drop. Action movies stimulate dopamine and testosterone for men, while talking, caring, and sharing movies stimulate serotonin and oxytocin for women. When movies have both ingredients, both men and women are drawn to them.

If a man has higher levels of testosterone, he can make the drive to the bridges of Madison County without falling asleep. Years later, with normal dopamine and testosterone levels, I can now easily make this drive and enjoy every minute of the way.

NEEDING TO SIT AT THE SHOPPING MALL

Another example of how women are energized by increasing oxytocin and relatively low testosterone levels and men are not comes from my experiences in shopping malls. When men shop, they tend to be very goal-oriented. If they go in for pants, they try to get out with pants in the shortest amount of time. If their objective is to find pants, they don't even think about getting matching shirts and shoes. This focused approach is very stimulating of testosterone. Women may go shopping for one thing, but they will also shop for a variety of other things in the process. Not only do they explore and discover more for themselves, but they will also be shopping for other people as well.

If she is not rushed in life, my wife can relax as she goes shopping. Thinking in a caring and sharing kind of manner produces healthy oxytocin, which increases levels of relaxation. If I tag along with her, I am done after about twenty minutes, while she stays energized. I am completely worn out. I rejoice when we go into a store and there is a chair for me to sit in while she is trying on dresses.

After about twenty minutes of shopping with a woman, the man is completely worn out and the woman is glowing.

There is a big distinction here. Women's stores have chairs for husbands to sit in, men's stores don't have chairs for women to sit in. This is because women don't need to sit when their husbands are trying on clothes. Even the thought of him wearing something new excites her levels of energy and well-being.

The activity of shopping, particularly if it includes shopping for others, is oxytocin-producing. When a man shops with and for his wife, he will wear out, because low testosterone results in low endorphins. When a woman shops with and for her husband, she will not wear out. Her higher oxytocin levels reward her with endorphins, and her low testosterone level doesn't reduce this high.

OXYTOCIN AND LASTING ROMANCE

Creating romance is one of the most powerful ways to balance our hormones. Oxytocin is the key to lasting romance. A woman doesn't feel in the mood unless she first feels stress-free. This is a big difference between men and women. Men can use physical intimacy as a way to lessen stress, but women get in the mood after their stress levels go down. For a man to feel attraction and desire, love is not necessarily a prerequisite. It will certainly enhance his experience, but it is not a requirement. For women, the love hormone oxytocin is the foundation upon which the house of romance can be built.

For romance to thrive, a woman needs to feel special. It is not enough that in a dire emergency a man would risk his life for her. Every day, in the midst of ordinary life, she needs to get messages that she is special. To focus a man's attention on what is required to meet this most important need, I have neatly summarized the solution. These ideas are more fully explained in my book *Men Are from Mars, Women Are from Venus.* Even if you read this book a while ago, it is time to read it again. After you have absorbed the new insights in this book, each sentence of *Men Are from Mars* will have new meaning. Here is a summary of what I said there on romance.

A woman needs to feel the assurance that she is still special to a man. In the beginning of a relationship, a man goes overboard to let her know that she is special. Once this message is communicated successfully, he mistakenly concludes that he doesn't have to give her this assurance anymore. This is far from the truth.

As she gets older, after the inevitable ups and downs of any relationship, she needs more assurance that after all these years her partner still loves her.

A man reasons that he doesn't have to remind her of his name every day, so why can't she just remember that he loves her?

Knowing his name and receiving assurance are two different worlds. They are as different as knowing what it is like to have sex with her and actually doing it. In a similar manner, the action of saying "I love you" actually stimulates an oxytocin response in her. This response needs to happen many times a day.

This is accomplished by using your mind and body in her presence to demonstrate these three kinds of love:

1. Caring
2. Understanding
3. Respect

These are the three magic keys. The fourth key is doing lots of little things, as opposed to one or two big demonstrations every week or month. To create lasting romance, demonstrate in *little* ways that you care, understand, and respect her. Focus on doing little things rather than big things.

Show in *little* ways that you care, understand, and respect her.

When women keep score, every act of love is equal. If you bring her a dozen roses you get one point. If you give her one rose you get one point. Instead of a dozen roses at one time, bring one rose twelve times. You do the math. That's right—you get twelve points for the price of one.

This example illustrates the whole secret of romance. It is doing little things on a consistent basis. When you remember to empty the trash without her having to remind you, you get bonus points.

BUILDING THE FIRE OF ROMANCE

Doing little things to create romance is like building a fire. You cannot start it with the big logs. You have to start it with some paper, then add kindling and the big logs. In the beginning of a relationship, we naturally start out with the paper and kindling. After we put the big logs in, we stop. The big logs are commitment, fidelity, and marriage.

When you build a fire, you have to start with kindling first.

To keep the passion alive in our relationships, we need to start out every day with paper and kindling as well. Here are a few examples of how to keep a woman's oxytocin levels high:

• When you get up in the morning, give her a hug. When you leave her in the morning for work, give her a good-bye hug. When you return home, find her and give her a hug, and *always* give her a hug before bed. Although this hug may just seem like kindling to a man, it is as important as the big logs.

Giving hugs is also a way a woman can raise her oxytocin levels. If he doesn't remember, then she can also initiate a hug.

• Asking her about her day is a way of saying you care and that you are interested. Even if you are not particularly interested in all the extra details—no man is—by being attentive, you let her know that you are interested in her and care about her happiness. Remember to just listen when she talks about her problems. She is not asking you to solve them.

If her partner doesn't ask about her day, then a wise woman initiates the conversation anyway. Instead of asking questions, she should just launch into telling him about her day.

• Whenever possible, offer to help. When a man literally uses his muscles, time, and energy in the presence of a woman to protect her and serve her needs, he is actively stimulating serotonin and oxytocin in her.

• When you come home from work, devote at least twenty minutes three times a week to spending quality time with her.

Try to remember some things from what goes on in your day so that she will feel more included in your day. A woman wants a man to be interested in her day, but she also wants to feel included in his.

When he gets home, it is best for a woman to make her first interaction a positive one. If she has a complaint, it is best to share it later. First impressions leave the biggest impression.

• Make sure to give at least one compliment a day. More is better. If she gets a haircut, make sure to compliment it. If she is wearing something new or just different, make sure to notice it and reassure her that she looks really great.

• Whenever you have the chance, touch her in an affectionate and not sexual manner. This keeps the oxytocin flowing.

She doesn't have to wait for the man's affectionate touches; she too can be affectionate, and he will appreciate and reciprocate.

When a woman doesn't get enough serotonin stimulated, she begins to feel like giving more is unfair because she doesn't get back. When she reaches the point of not being motivated to give, rather than complain or ask for more, try speaking her language. The act of giving to her will make it safe for her to give back to you. As her serotonin levels rise, she will then be happy to give more again.

ALONE IN THE WOODS

A woman greatly appreciates coming home to a man who can help lift her from the stress of her day. When her oxytocin levels drop, due to too much testosterone activity, the increasing serotonin and oxytocin of a loving and supportive relationship can assist her. The most potent stress-reducing activity for a woman is romance. Romance doesn't always mean "Let's head for the bedroom." From a woman's perspective, when a man helps out doing the dishes after dinner, this is romantic. All the little things that say I care are the kindling for building the fire of romance.

While the little ways of supporting are the basis of building the fires of romance, to keep it going, you also need the big logs. The big logs in this example are romantic dates and getaways. These are essential for romance to thrive. Even with the easy-to-burn foreplay of good communication and the kindling of helping her and sharing domestic responsibilities, the big logs of romantic dates are essential.

On a romantic date or getaway, the man is protecting and serving the woman in a manner that says she is special to him. This helps give her the feeling that her needs will be met. This stimulates in her the feelings of increased serotonin. She feels content, comforted, and optimistic. This makes it safe for her to give of herself, which leads to rising oxytocin levels. As her hormones increase, her passion gradually builds.

Her body responds to his actions with increased appreciation, acceptance, and trust. Intellectually she may appreciate, accept, and trust him, but this is different from actually stimulating the hormones of these feelings in her body. At these special times he should do most of the dopamine and testosterone activities, and she the serotonin and oxytocin activities. Here is an example to illustrate this point.

Imagine going on a romantic getaway in the woods. You are in a cabin with your romantic partner. After the sun sets, it is very dark and quiet. The fire is burning and the mood is set for a romantic evening. Then you both hear a noise. It's a little scary, since you are way out in the woods late at night. It could be a big black bear that is stalking you. Maybe it is an intruder. The noise happens again, but this time it is a little louder. You realize that somebody needs to go outside and find out what is happening.

Imagine that he says, "Honey, I am scared. Would you go out and see what is making that noise? I will sit by the phone and call for help if you call out or don't come back."

She goes out to see what the noise is all about. It is just a raccoon getting into the trash cans. When she returns and tells him that everything is all right, he says, "Thanks so much for going out there in the dark and checking it out. I am still a little scared. Would you just hold me for a while?"

When she holds him, what are the feelings that come up in her? Suddenly she will feel protective (Mars) and mothering (Venus) toward him. She will have a good dose of both testosterone and oxytocin, but her serotonin levels will be low because she doesn't feel that she has someone she can depend on in times of danger. Taking a risk on her own outside has raised her dopamine levels but lowered her serotonin levels. Will she feel romantic that night? I think not. She certainly feels loving, but it is not romantic.

Now let's turn the tables. There is a noise outside in the dark and she says, "Honey, I am scared. Would you go out and see what is making that noise? I will sit by the phone and call for help if you don't come back." He goes out to see what the noise is all about. It is just a raccoon in the trash cans. If he is wise, he takes a little longer to build the suspense. When he returns and tells her that everything is all right, she says, "Thanks so much for checking it out. I am still a little scared. Would you just hold me for a while?"

Now he holds her for a while. What do you think is going to happen that night? For sure they will have one of the most romantic evenings in their relationship.

Why? Because of the romantic hormones that were produced. By going outside to protect and serve her, he found his testosterone and dopamine levels went way up. By risking his life for her, he experienced increased dopamine (energy, strength, and pleasure). By trusting and depending on him, she felt her serotonin levels go way up. This increased trust and comfort created the safety to freely give of herself to him. Her oxytocin levels rose and her heart opened even more.

Now let's add one more element. Let's say he had a broken foot and couldn't go out. The fact that he would if he could will also stimulate testosterone in him and serotonin in her as long as he doesn't ask *her* to hold him. After she returns, if she is still shaking and he listens to her and holds her, all the right hormones get stimulated. In this case, she feels he is there and doing his best to help. As long as a man is not too needy, that is all women require for increasing serotonin and oxytocin.

KEEPING THE FIRES OF PASSION BURNING

To keep the fires of passion burning in both himself and his partner, a man needs to take charge and make sure that his partner gets the support she needs. If a man forgets to take on this job, it is a mistake for a woman to wait. She should take charge just as she would at work, but in this case she should take charge and delegate the responsibility to him. This means she needs to make the request for him to follow through and do the deed.

In making this request, she needs to be specific. It doesn't work to complain that she is not happy or that he is not romantic. She shouldn't say, "Just surprise me with something romantic." Instead, she must spell it out in the least number of words in terms of a request.

For example, she could say, "Let's get away next weekend. I have time open, and I noticed on your calendar that you didn't have much planned. I would like to go to the Auberge du Soleil in Napa. Let's stay for two nights this time. I love their restaurant. We could eat there, and we could eat in town the other night. Would you make reservations?"

By being specific, she helps motivate him. Men need a little kindling as well. By asking for what she wants in positive and specific terms, she does her part to create lasting romance.

Women today are hungry for romance because working in a testosterone-oriented job lowers their Venusian hormone levels. Romance and everything it entails increases serotonin and oxytocin, which then increases a woman's endorphins. To cope with the stress of work and life, women commonly turn to romantic novels, self-help books, fashion magazines, gossip magazines, comfort foods such as fried foods, desserts, and chocolate, and TV talk shows. Anything that involves romance, relationships, parenting, children, homes, weddings, dieting, eating, restaurants, recipes, gardening, communication, shopping, makeup, and fashion helps to stimulate serotonin and oxytocin.

At the top of their list, women are looking for romance. Men often conclude that if a woman can provide for herself, she doesn't need him. With new insight about a woman's need for romance, a man realizes that he has the power to provide something she can't get on her own. He is needed much more than he thought. There is a big problem out there, and he is the solution. Men are needed and wanted.

Men are often not romantic because they don't even know what it means. Romance is not so important to men. They may complain about not enough sex, but rarely does a man think in terms of not enough romance. Romance is the great stimulator of serotonin and oxytocin. Men aren't searching for those hormones. Sex is a different matter. Men are preoccupied with sex because it produces testosterone, dopamine, and plenty of endorphins.

By taking the time to learn about our different emotional needs and by doing what it takes to feed and exercise our bodies properly, both men and women can begin making their dreams come true. If we continue to live in ignorance, then nothing can change. Even if we have taken the time to study and educate ourselves, we need a diet and exercise plan we can and will stick to in order to put into action all that we have learned. It is time for a change. With this powerful insight on reducing stress through improving our relationship skills, we are now ready to focus on feeding our bodies and brains the raw materials to create the right hormones and neural transmitters. With *The Mars and Venus Diet and Exercise Solution,* you can now begin creating the brain chemistry of health, happiness, and lasting romance.

8

SAY GOOD-BYE TO DIETING

In order to learn how to eat and supplement your diet to create healthy chemistry, you first need to know why dieting doesn't work. As you say good-bye to dieting, you will lay the foundation for producing the brain chemistry to improve your relationships and increase your health and happiness. If you are overweight, one of the wonderful side effects is immediate weight loss.

When popular reduction diets require eating less, they often fail. They can't work because everything in life is about balance. What goes up comes down. Eating less eventually results in eating more. It is that simple. Not only will eating more cause weight gain for some, but more important, it will inhibit the production of necessary brain chemicals.

In the short term, as an act of will, you can deprive yourself of the food you want to eat, but later, when the pendulum swings in the other direction, you will want to overeat. Even if you are highly motivated for health reasons, you will always be battling with unpleasant cravings for foods you can't or shouldn't eat. This is not the way we are supposed to live our lives. Research reveals that almost all women struggle daily with unhealthy food cravings.

Unless we are highly motivated by a serious health condition, diet programs that require a lot of willpower are hard to adhere to. Applying willpower for a diet is like having to lift a heavy weight. At a certain point, you need to rest, and there goes the diet plan. A lasting food program must be easy to follow and delicious, too.

Applying willpower for a diet is like carrying a heavy weight all the time.

With *The Mars and Venus Diet and Exercise Solution,* you can say good-bye to deprivation diets and willpower. By following this plan for a short period of time, you create healthy brain chemistry by eating what you want and how much you want.

What's the catch?

The catch is your desires will change. When your diet stimulates balanced brain chemicals, healthy food tastes better. When your cells are being properly nourished, you don't feel the need to overeat. What you want to eat and how much you want to eat changes in nine days when your cells are not starving and each day your body is producing healthy brain chemicals.

What you want to eat changes in nine days when your brain is balanced and your cells are not starving.

THE THREE GUIDELINES

The Mars and Venus Solution works because the three basic guidelines are easy to follow. Anyone can do it and continue doing it. Give it a try for two weeks and you will never want to give it up. For this program to work, I will give you many suggestions and pointers, but there are three essential guidelines to follow:

1. **You eat at least three meals a day.** Women, who are more prone to problems with low blood sugar, need to eat three meals a day and at least two snacks. In this diet plan, less is not better. More is better, and definitely more of the healthy foods you enjoy most. At each meal, you eat an almost equal proportion of calories from each of the three main nutrient groups: proteins, carbohydrates, and dietary fat. The right balance for you may vary according to your body type, weight, level of exercise, mental state, and, most important, your gender. You will find more information on this in Chapters 9, 10, and 11.

2. **You follow the Mars and Venus breathing, bouncing, and exercise routine for at least ten to thirty minutes when you first wake up.**

3. **You replace your breakfast with a low-calorie, highly nutritious breakfast shake.** All the necessary ingredients can be found at your local health food store. Once you have regained your ideal weight you can occasionally include a normal breakfast with your morning shake if you wish.

That's all there is to it. In the next five chapters, we will explore in great detail what to do and why it works. Understanding the importance of each of these steps gives you the motivation to follow the program. After understanding the principles behind the program, you will want to follow it, because it makes sense to you and *you* think it is a good idea.

FINDING BALANCE IN YOUR DIET

Everything in life and in your diet is about balance. If you cut back on calories, eating less than your body needs, then eventually you will swing the other way, feeling a need to consume more calories than you need. This is commonly called yo-yo dieting. You eat less for a time only to binge and overeat later. Each time you eat less, you go out of balance, and the cycle repeats. Each time the cycle repeats, both men and women tend to gain back a little more weight. Without the Mars and Venus

Solution, you find it increasingly difficult to get back to your ideal weight and stay there.

Eating less almost always results in eating too much later.

Even healthy diets generally don't work, because unhealthy people don't want to eat healthy food. When you are not healthy, wholesome food doesn't even taste good; junk food tastes good. Let's define junk food to be any processed food that is nutritionally deficient. We will list them in Chapter 11.

When your brain chemistry is not balanced, your mind and body will crave nutritionally deficient foods. When you eat junk, you want more junk. On the other hand, if you are getting the nutrients that your body and brain require, your tastes change. You begin to enjoy the taste of healthy foods.

When you are unhealthy, you will crave junk food.

Your brain determines what you like. If a food produces dopamine for a dopamine-deficient man, he will begin to like that food more within nine days. When a food produces serotonin for a serotonin-deficient woman, she will begin to hunger for it within nine days.

WOMEN AND CHOCOLATE

Chocolate is a prime example. At the onset of a woman's period, her serotonin levels fall and her mood echoes that fall. She begins to crave chocolate, that magic food. Chocolate produces an instant but temporary surge in serotonin levels. As a result, her taste for chocolate is magnified.

While most commercial chocolate is filled with chemicals and additives and can be nutrient-deficient, more expensive or higher quality brands are made with pure and healthy ingredients. My favorite brand of chocolate and a favorite of the Venusians at my house are Tamera Truffles (www.e3livealgae.com/chocolate/). These chocolates contain 100 percent organic ingredients, including organic dark Belgian chocolate, fresh organic cream, organic vanilla, and dried cane juice for sweetness. They are filled with powerful antioxidants, chlorophyll, and other healthy ingredients. Each chocolate also contains 500 milligrams of healthy bluegreen algae for extra protein.

Popular health bars covered in chocolate are among the easiest ways to get your children to eat healthy vitamin supplements. These little treats make a great snack and even create a healthy balance of protein, fat, and carbohydrate. They are particularly good for women and girls.

There are good reasons why giving chocolate to a woman was and will always be romantic. Moderate amounts of chocolate have been proven to stimulate brain balance so that serotonin and oxytocin levels go up and stress is dramatically reduced. Every woman needs to have a backup stash of healthy and nutritious chocolate to help her through the difficult times. Chocolate is filled with healthy properties. Chocolate itself is not a problem—too much refined sugar is. Moderation is the solution.

IDENTIFYING AND HEALING FOOD ALLERGIES

Often if you eat too much of a particular food or you eat it in quantities that exceed what you need, your body will begin to reject those foods; you will become allergic to them. The most common food allergies are to dairy products, sugar, soy, eggs, and bread. Some of the symptoms of food allergies are excess mucus in your sinuses, nasal passages, and throat; high blood sugar; fatigue and brain fog; headaches; colds; physical discomfort; and constipation and gas. Food allergies make you more vulnerable to hay fever, asthma, or allergies to mold or dust.

The biggest problem with food allergies is that we crave the foods to which we are allergic. This causes us to eat way too much of them, which then intensifies our food allergies. A Mars and Venus diet takes away your cravings by balancing brain chemistry and feeding the cells. When we feed our cells the nutrients they need and stop overeating, many of the symptoms of food allergies disappear.

If you have food allergies, the easiest way to discover what you are allergic to is to observe what foods you eat most. If you love cookies, then you are allergic to something in the cookies. Probably you are allergic to everything in the cookie: refined sugar and flour as well as the butter and milk.

If you are allergic to cookies, when you are hungry, all you want is cookies!

With healthy brain chemistry, your cravings for foods decrease, and you will feel free to eat a varied diet with different foods every day. As you begin to eat a more balanced diet with nutrient-dense foods for breakfast, food allergies have less of an effect.

Sometimes just by eating the right balance of carbohydrates, proteins, and fats, your food allergy will disappear. For example, you may be allergic to cheese, but when it is combined with whole wheat bread and a tomato, for some people, the allergy temporarily disappears. Combining foods in a healthy manner makes them much more appealing to your body. In Chapters 9, 10, and 11, we will explore the importance of combining protein, fats, and carbohydrates at every meal.

You can also become allergic to your partner in a marriage, from too much time spent together without a balance of time alone, time with friends, and time together with friends. Couples who don't socialize with other couples or take alone time can easily become bored, annoyed, or irritated with each other. The annoyance generated by too much time together tends to go away very quickly in a social situation, when the couple is getting the other social or emotional nutrients they need.

A HAPPY MIND THINKS HAPPY THOUGHTS

Have you ever noticed that when you are in a good mood you think happy thoughts, and when you are in a bad mood you think negative thoughts? It is the same with your body. When your body is feeling healthy and nourished, it wants only healthy food. But when it is not healthy or it is undernourished, your body craves unhealthy food.

A happy mind automatically thinks happy
thoughts, and a healthy body automatically
hungers for healthful foods.

Another way to determine which foods are really not very good for your body is to notice what you want when you are feeling upset. Emotionally upset people almost always crave foods that are not good for them. Happy, relaxed, and satisfied persons will tend to like healthier food. At the very least, they will have much more control over what they eat.

I know there are very spartan people who clearly eat to live rather than live to eat, but I think life should be a combination of both approaches to food. I eat to live, but I also live to eat. I look forward to eating my food, and lots of it. To achieve this balance, I just needed to apply enough willpower at the beginning of the program to exercise for thirty minutes and eat a healthy, balanced breakfast. As you will soon discover, that's all it takes.

FINDING YOUR NORTH STAR

If you want to arrive at a destination, you need a reference point that lets you know when you are on track and when you are not. To achieve any goal, we need feedback as to what is working and what is not. If you are trying to navigate a plane or boat, you need a compass to let you know where you are on course and to help you reset your course if necessary.

In the old days, before compasses, navigators would use the North Star for this necessary feedback. By referencing your position with the North Star, you could always determine what direction to take. When it comes to finding the best diet, you have your own personal North Star. Your body gives you the perfect feedback regarding what to eat and how much. But you have to listen carefully to its signals.

Your body gives you the perfect feedback regarding what to eat and how much.

Your body may be saying one thing, but you hear something else. Here are some examples of not listening to what your body is telling you:

- Your body is saying "Give me water," and you reach for a soft drink.
- Your body is saying "I am sleepy, give me stimulating exercise so I can wake up," and you hear "I am sleepy," and sleep more.
- Your body is saying that this cookie with refined sugar is not nutritious enough, and you hear "One cookie is not enough, eat more."
- Your body is saying "This meal is mineral- and enzyme-deficient, give me supplements," and you hear "This meal is not enough, eat more."

As you begin to supplement and balance your diet with the nutrients that you need to create healthy brain chemistry, you will begin to live in the zone of endless energy, unconditional happiness, and unlimited love most of the time. Using this normal state of mind as your reference point, you will correctly interpret your body's messages. You will know what works for your body and brain and what doesn't.

MOTIVATION TO EAT GOOD FOODS

When you know what a balanced state feels like, you can tell if a food causes you to fall out of the zone. I am personally motivated to eat healthy food for two reasons. First, my tastes have changed, and most of the time I find that healthy food tastes much better. The second reason is the feedback I get from my body. If I don't eat right, I instantly go out of the zone. When you put your finger in a fire, your body learns very quickly not to do that again.

Likewise, when your meal suddenly saps your energy instead of raising it, you will feel the need to get the right foods in the right amounts for you. By listening to your body, you are freed from having to follow the conflicting advice of experts.

By listening to your body, you are freed from
having to follow the conflicting advice of experts.

When I do eat junk food, I will supplement that meal with extra minerals, vitamins, and enzymes. This minimizes the negative effect of junk food. The next day I might do the Mars and Venus cleansing routine. Junk food not only throws your body out of balance but gives your body more toxins to deal with.

When you consume the proper nutrients, your body functions like a well-oiled engine. Eating junk food is toxic. If someone were to put dirt in your car oil, you would drain the oil before adding more. With this program, you will start the day with exercises to stimulate your metabolism and cleanse the toxins from your body.

Each person is unique, with different tastes and preferences, so there is no perfect diet plan for everyone. Eventually you will determine all the right foods for you. When you are getting immediate feedback from your body, it becomes easy to determine the best guidelines and follow them.

This program will help you to get to peak experience and stay there long enough so that you can then determine what works and what doesn't. By following the precise breakfast guidelines after a minimum of ten to thirty minutes of special exercise, you will start your day with balanced brain cleansing; after that, you will be better equipped to determine the best foods for you.

WHY PEOPLE SKIP BREAKFAST

Many people skip breakfast. This lowers your metabolism and sets you up to overeat later. When you skip breakfast, you may get a lot of short-term energy, but when you finally do eat, you will crave the wrong foods. By eating a balanced breakfast, you will have an active metabolism that can burn fat efficiently, build lean body mass, and most important, keep your brain chemicals balanced.

Missing breakfast lowers your metabolism and sets you up to overeat later.

The most common reason we skip breakfast is that we are too busy. We have time for others around us, but not enough time to nourish ourselves. In our crowded lives, there is just so much to do.

Many people skip breakfast because it feels good. If they did eat breakfast they would experience a drop in energy. Instead, they have coffee or tea and maybe a pastry. I have skipped breakfast for most of my life. I didn't like eating in the morning because it sapped me of my strength, clarity, and energy. I was eating the wrong foods, foods that were nutritionally deficient.

People often skip breakfast because they think it might help with weight management. As we pass forty and the weight starts building around the waist, many people figure missing a meal is probably a good thing; it might help them lose weight, or at least prevent weight gain. This is not the case. It does just the opposite.

When you miss breakfast, your body concludes that there is

not a lot of fuel available, and so it turns down the metabolism. Not only do you have less energy, but it is also harder to burn excess body fat. When the body thinks there is not enough food, it starts holding on to what it has got.

When the body thinks there is not enough food, it starts holding on to what it has got.

Think of your body as an old-fashioned steam engine. To fuel the engine, you need to feed the fire with coal. When there is no coal available, the stoker slows down so that all the available fuel is not consumed. Likewise, your metabolism slows down for the rest of the day when you don't eat breakfast.

I remember driving in my car late one night on Highway 1 between Santa Cruz and San Francisco. There is a dark and lonely stretch of highway along the coast for about thirty miles. After ten miles along that route, I realized that my gas tank was almost empty. To conserve gas and make it last, I slowed way down. I did eventually get to a gas station, but it took a long time. In a similar way, when your body doesn't eat for a few hours, it assumes there is no fuel available, and the metabolism slows down to avoid running out of fuel completely.

When you eat breakfast, your body gets a clear message that it can get energy, and the metabolism is then set for the day. With the right amount of food for breakfast, you will be activating your metabolism to burn the calories you eat and produce the brain chemicals you need. You want to burn all the calories you eat so that your body doesn't store extra calories as fat. Undigested foods become toxic in your body.

THE IMPORTANCE OF ENZYMES

One reason people skip breakfast is that our breakfast foods are deficient in minerals and enzymes. Whenever you cook or process food with heat, it kills *all* the enzymes. Enzymes activate the digestion and assimilation process in the body. When your food has no enzymes, your pancreas has to produce the enzymes necessary to digest your food. The pancreas must shift from making the metabolic enzymes necessary to produce healthy brain chemicals. To digest your enzyme-deficient food, your body stops producing healthy chemicals. Everyone knows that we need enzymes to digest, but we also need thousands of other enzymes to regulate the many metabolic processes besides digestion.

When we eat an enzyme-deficient breakfast, the production of metabolic enzymes is blocked, and the necessary brain chemicals like dopamine and serotonin are not produced in adequate supplies. The result of eating a nutrient-deficient breakfast is to feel tired and sluggish a little later.

People with low metabolism will rarely skip breakfast because they require food right away in the morning. When they get up, they need to eat! By eating cooked or processed food in the morning, they inhibit the pancreas from producing the metabolic enzymes to produce brain chemistry. For these people, it is better to do thirty minutes of exercise to raise their metabolism, and then to eat. If they are overweight, it is best to replace breakfast with a shake until they are back to normal. After their normal weight is reached, it is fine to eat breakfast again, after they have taken their shake. In Chapter 9, I will provide you with a complete list of the specific ingredients to produce balanced brain chemistry.

People with high metabolism enjoy missing breakfast because they easily burn the stored energy in the liver and experience the benefit of metabolic enzymes producing dopamine and serotonin.

Eating a nutrient-deficient breakfast can make people sluggish and tired.

To avoid feeling tired in the morning, the people with high metabolisms just skip breakfast. Eventually they run low on energy and need to eat. Skipping breakfast—or any meal, for that matter—is one of the primary reasons we crave unhealthy food and eat too much food in one sitting. We skip a meal and then overeat at the next meal because we are starving.

THE SEROTONIN EFFECT

Skipping breakfast is more devastating to women than men, because morning is the most important time for the production of serotonin. Our eyes are more sensitive to light in the morning. The morning light stimulates the pineal gland to begin producing serotonin. Yet to produce serotonin, the body needs the nourishment provided by amino acids.

We produce most of our serotonin supplies in the morning.

Amino acids are contained in the protein we eat. Protein in the morning is essential for producing serotonin, but too much protein will inhibit serotonin production in women. More protein creates dopamine for men. This difference is directly related to a man's higher muscle-to-fat ratio. Understanding how brain chemicals are affected by protein and exercise is one of the most important keys to balancing brain chemistry. Let's explore this relationship.

Brain chemicals are affected directly by our muscle-to-fat ratio.

Amino acids come from the proteins that we eat. The amino acid tryptophan is converted by the brain into serotonin. The amino acids phenylalanine and tyrosine are converted by the brain into dopamine. To create balanced brain chemistry, men and women need both serotonin and dopamine. As we have already established, men tend to be deficient in dopamine and women deficient in serotonin.

For brain chemicals to be produced, amino acids must first be transported through the brain-blood barrier. The brain-blood barrier protects the brain from toxic intruders and other harmful influences that might easily get into the blood from the stomach. As a result, amino acids have limited access to the brain. Tryptophan has to compete with all the other amino acids seeking transport through the brain-blood barrier. Being the smallest of the amino acids, it is the last to get through. If the overall amino acid count is very high, the brain absorbs less tryptophan to produce serotonin with. This is called the serotonin effect.

Amino acids are used not only by the brain but by the muscles as well. When we use our muscles, all of the amino acids except tryptophan are directed to the muscles. The muscles do not need tryptophan. When muscles are exercised, they absorb most of the amino acids, leaving no competition for tryptophan to cross the brain-blood barrier. Exercise directs competing amino acids to the muscles, and tryptophan is then easily absorbed by the brain.

Exercise directs competing amino acids to the muscles, and tryptophan is then easily absorbed by the brain.

This explains why men have higher levels of serotonin. They are born with a high muscle-to-fat ratio. When men eat protein, more of the amino acids are absorbed by the muscles, leaving tryptophan to be converted into serotonin. If a woman is not exercising, eating protein will cause her dopamine levels to go up and her serotonin levels to go down, because she has less muscle and more fat.

Men who do not get enough protein become dopamine-deficient. If a woman eats too much protein, there are so many competing amino acids that her tryptophan does not get converted into serotonin. Even with enough protein, men tend to be dopamine-deficient because a higher muscle mass can direct the amino acids phenylalanine and tyrosine to the muscles and not to the brain.

As long as a man or woman is eating a nutritious balance of nutrients, both dopamine and serotonin can be produced in the right amounts. Women have to be particularly careful not to overeat protein in the morning and to get plenty of exercise before breakfast. After exercise, the muscles require all the amino acids to be restored, freeing up an abundance of tryptophan in the brain.

For a woman, the morning is the most important time of the day to generate serotonin. By skipping breakfast, she does get the benefit of metabolic enzymes, but the effect will still be limited because she has not eaten any protein, fat, or carbohydrate. The best solution for her is to take a balanced breakfast shake that will support the maximum production of serotonin. Extreme dieting and skipping breakfast are the worst things a woman can do.

In addition to the amino acids provided by protein, a woman needs to consume enough fat for the production of serotonin. A high-protein diet doesn't work and neither does a low-fat diet. Brain chemicals are regulated by prostaglandins, which are created by the essential fatty acids found in dietary fat. Essential fatty acids (EFAs) are the building blocks of dietary fat and oils. These EFAs are required for the production of brain chemicals. The two most important EFAs are omega-3 and omega-6. Our common diet has too much omega-6 and not enough omega-3. Omega-3 fatty acids are essential for the processing of serotonin. The right balance of fat and protein is essential for brain chemistry for both men and women.

A high-carbohydrate breakfast will stimulate serotonin production, but too much will make blood sugar unstable. Unstable blood sugar eventually inhibits the production of serotonin. When excess sugar enters the bloodstream, insulin is released, directing all the amino acids to the muscles except L-tryptophan, which is then easily absorbed by the brain and converted into serotonin. By eating refined sugars, a woman gets the benefit of increased serotonin, but when her blood sugar drops quickly, so does the serotonin production.

Eating doughnuts or other high-sugar breakfast treats creates a temporary surge in serotonin.

Many serotonin diets recommend eating more carbohydrates in the morning. This is very effective as long as the insulin release is not so great that blood sugar becomes unstable. By balancing fat, protein, and carbohydrate, a woman can get exactly the right formula for her to create maximum serotonin.

A similar formula works for men. Men just require more protein and women require more dietary fat rich in omega-3s. Both require enough carbohydrates to fuel the brain with the sugar it needs to function. The Mars and Venus blended shake solution takes these gender differences into account.

DEHYDRATION AND CELLULAR STARVATION

Some people become uneasy with the thought of skipping breakfast and having a shake instead. The thought of missing a meal seems scary and unhealthy. Having the Mars and Venus shake every morning does not mean you are missing a meal. You are replacing your normal breakfast, which is nutritionally deficient, with a shake containing all the nutrients necessary for breakfast. It will not have the sentimental value of eggs and bacon or blueberry pancakes, but it is much healthier.

There are two reasons we feel a need to overeat or are reluctant not to eat a regular meal. The first is dehydration, and the second is mineral deficiency. Water is required by the body to deliver nutrients to the cells. When our bodies are dehydrated, without adequate water, our cells are starving. You may be eating plenty of nutrients, but they are not getting to the cells. Besides needing water to deliver nutrients, the body also requires water to clean out toxins. Without an abundance of water in the body to remove excess toxins, the cells can be poisoned. Without water, the cells cannot release the waste products of metabolism.

Besides needing water to deliver nutrients, the body also requires water to clean out toxins.

Water is nature's miracle cleanser. It is essential for the lymphatic system to clean your body. Unless you drink enough water, your body's lymphatic system cannot clean away all the toxins you ingest and breathe in as well as the normal toxic by-products of healthy metabolism. There are books solely about the many health benefits of water. My favorite is *Your Body's Many Cries for Water* by Fereydoor Batmanghelidj, M.D. Almost all sickness and many of the undesirable symptoms of aging have been directly linked to chronic dehydration. A child is 70 percent water and an average seventy-year-old is 30 percent water.

Most people over fifty are dehydrated. They just don't drink enough water. Without water, we will die in a few weeks. Water is essential not only for cleansing but for delivering nutrients to the cells. Most people are literally dying of thirst, and they don't know it.

Water is essential for cleansing and for delivering nutrients to the cells.

Even water retention is a symptom of dehydration. The body holds on to water because the cells are not getting enough. Not enough good fats in your diet will block your body's ability to assimilate water at a cellular level.

Many people don't drink enough water because they have to urinate all the time. Frequent urination is another sign of dehydration. It means the water is just passing through, not being assimilated by the cells and tissues. Think of the body as a sponge. When it is dry, it cannot absorb water. When a sponge becomes saturated with water, you can squeeze out all the water and it will quickly absorb more.

Frequent urination is another sign of dehydration.

It can take many months of adequate water supply to become fully hydrated. It is not just a matter of drinking enough water in a day. It takes years to become dehydrated, and it can take many months to hydrate again. By adding trace minerals to your water, you will become hydrated much faster. In Chapter 9, we explore a morning drink that efficiently hydrates your body.

Drinking water doesn't always increase hydration. What you put in that water determines what your body does with it. If you drink water with caffeine, then that water doesn't count toward your daily need. The caffeine in coffee, tea, and soft drinks is a diuretic. Diuretics prevent your body from assimilating water. What goes in will immediately flow out. By drinking lots of stimulants, you may be ingesting a lot of water, but the end result is dehydration.

Alcoholic beverages are also diuretics. People suffer from hangovers not from the alcohol consumed but from the dehydration that has occurred. By drinking more water with your stimulants or alcohol, you will have less dehydration.

If you drink water with caffeine, that water doesn't count toward your daily need.

Without sufficient water, the lymphatic system cannot operate, and the liver takes over as an emergency measure. To take over this job, the liver stops processing amino acids for the production of dopamine and serotonin. An underactive lymphatic system inhibits the production of healthy brain chemicals.

An underactive lymphatic system inhibits the production of serotonin and dopamine.

A toxic liver is also linked to an imbalance in the thyroid gland, which in turn controls the burning or storing of excess fat. Proper functioning of the liver to process amino acids is essential for normal functioning of the thyroid gland and weight management. Many people who have difficulty losing weight have an imbalance in thyroid functioning. With a more active lymphatic system supplemented by plenty of water, the thyroid gland can function as it is designed to.

With a more active lymphatic system, the thyroid gland can function better.

One of the ways the liver deals with excess toxins is to increase body fat to enfold these toxins and to protect the body from their influence. This process is primarily responsible for what is commonly called liver gut. To protect the body from toxins, the liver triggers fat production in the gut to store the toxins. This toxic buildup causes that bulge so many people get at the waistline as they get older.

Practically no amount of exercise will make liver gut go away. This is a job for the lymphatic system. Once you begin activating your lymphatic system with sufficient oxygen, water, and movement in the morning, your liver can remove your liver gut.

With sufficient oxygen, water, and movement in the morning, your liver can remove excess weight around the waist.

The morning is the most important time for liver cleansing. This is talked about extensively in the five-thousand-year-old Chinese system of medicine. According to this system, the body focuses on different organs throughout the night. In the morning, during the two hours right before dawn, the body has the most energy available for the liver. This is the best time to do lymph-stimulating exercises. Stimulating the lymphatic system lightens the load for your liver so it can do its other work and produce neural transmitters. Modern research has gone on to confirm the importance of the early morning hours around sunrise to stimulate the production of serotonin.

Stimulating the lymphatic system lightens the load for your liver, so it can produce healthy brain chemistry.

Most nutritionists agree that your body requires about 64 ounces of water a day when you are healthy. This means eight 8-ounce glasses. If you are overweight, sick, or tired, you will need even more.

All sickness is linked to toxic buildup in the body. By starting your day with a glass of water to stimulate your lymphatic system, you are taking your first and most important step to creating the brain chemistry of health, happiness, and lasting romance. Without the water, nothing else can work.

To determine your minimum water requirements, divide your weight in pounds by two; that is the number of ounces of pure water you need in a day. If you weigh 128 pounds, you need 64 ounces, or eight glasses a day. If you weigh 196 pounds, you need 98 ounces, or twelve glasses a day. The water in juice and soup also counts to satisfy your body's need for H_2O.

In order to consume enough water, keep in mind that coffee, black tea, soft drinks, and alcoholic drinks will dehydrate your body. If you are going to drink these substances, always supplement your body with another glass of water above and beyond your normal requirement for every serving. Decaffeinated coffee still has half the diuretic effect of normal coffee.

Coffee, black tea, soft drinks, and alcoholic drinks dehydrate your body.

If you exercise and work up a sweat, you will also need more water. Hundreds of people have found that with *The Mars and*

Venus Diet and Exercise Solution, they no longer need coffee for energy or alcohol to relax and have a good time. They may use these beverages occasionally as a social icebreaker or as a treat, but they are not dependent on them.

MINERAL DEFICIENCY

Our cells are starving and our brains are not producing healthy brain chemistry because the foods we eat are deficient in minerals. No matter how well you select the right foods for yourself, it will not be satisfying and you will want to overeat. This is so because everything you buy from the produce department of your grocery store is deficient in trace minerals.

> Everything you buy from the produce department of your grocery store is deficient in trace minerals.

Organic food products have a higher mineral content, but the level of these minerals is not even close to what it used to be just fifty years ago. An organic tomato in the grocery today has 50 percent fewer minerals than a regular store tomato of fifty years ago. Even with plenty of water, we can't get what we need, because the fresh produce is mineral-deficient and almost all of the processed food is stripped of its natural mineral content.

> An organic tomato in the grocery today has 50 percent fewer minerals than a regular store tomato of fifty years ago.

More than seventy years ago, the government issued a report acknowledging that farming practices in America had stripped the soil of minerals and that all foods were thus mineral-deficient. This announcement led to the beginning of the health food supplement business. Suddenly everyone recognized the need for mineral supplementation.

Although there was no awareness that trace minerals were absolutely essential for the production of healthy brain functioning, people did recognize that minerals were important for strong bones and physical health. Even with this increased awareness, the incidence of osteoporosis in women has skyrocketed. Not only are the foods we eat deficient in minerals, but the refined sugar we eat leaches out the small amount of minerals we store in our bones.

Mineral deficiency has greater repercussions than just causing weak bones or cavities in our teeth, though these are certainly significant problems. Mineral deficiency affects every aspect of our physical and mental health.

Mineral deficiency affects every aspect of our physical and mental health.

We already know the importance of vitamins. What is not as well-known but has been extensively researched is that vitamins cannot be assimilated without the aid of minerals. All tissues and internal fluids of our body contain varying quantities of minerals. Minerals are the constituents of bones, teeth, soft tissue, muscle, blood, and nerve cells.

Minerals are vital to our overall mental and physical well-being. They act as catalysts for the many biological and electrical reactions within the body, for muscle response, for the transmission of messages and energy through the nervous system, for the production of hormones, for digestion, and for the utilization of nutrients in foods.

Minerals have both structural and functional roles. They are components of body tissues and fluids and work in combination with enzymes, hormones, vitamins, and transport substances. The presence of trace minerals works as a factor to synthesize the production of brain chemicals.

Dr. Linus Pauling, twice the winner of a Nobel Prize, said, "You can trace every sickness, every disease, and every ailment to a mineral deficiency." Most of the problems we suffer today began with the mineral-deficient land our food is grown on and the animals that eat that produce.

Every sickness, every disease, and every ailment can be traced to a mineral deficiency.

When farmers discovered the quick results produced by artificial fertilizers at the beginning of last century, crop yields increased but the soil received only three nutrients, not the seventy-seven minerals and trace minerals found in the land before these nitrogen-based fertilizers were used. Within ten years, the land became mineral-deficient, incapable of producing crops with a balanced supply of minerals.

With the supplementation of nitrates, phosphates, and potassium, plants are able to flourish temporarily. For about ten years, they assimilate the minerals from the soil more easily. Without replenishing the ground with the seventy-seven minerals and trace minerals, farmers can still produce a crop yield, but the plants are mineral-deficient.

Here are a few more quotes to reinforce the reality of mineral deficiency and the importance of mineral supplementation.

- In 1912, Nobel Prize winner Dr. Alexis Carrel forecast that "Minerals in the soil control the metabolism in plants, animals, and man. All of life will either be healthy or unhealthy according to the fertility of the soil."
- In 1936, the U.S. Senate issued Document no. 264, which included the following warning: "The alarming fact is that foods (fruits, vegetables, and grains) now being raised on millions of acres of land that no longer contains enough of certain minerals are starving us—no matter how much of them we eat. No man of today can eat enough fruits and vegetables to supply his system with the minerals he requires for perfect health because his stomach isn't big enough to hold them."
- In 1988, the Surgeon General's Report on Health and Nutrition concluded that fifteen out of every twenty-one deaths in

the United States involved nutritional deficiencies (almost 75 percent).

• In 1992, world leaders concluded in the Earth Summit Report that over the past ten years, mineral depletion of the soil was over 76 percent in Europe and over 80 percent in America.

• In 1994, the U.S. Congress decisively concluded that ingestion of the proper nutrients actually prevents chronic disease.

Without nitrogen fertilizers, plants are dependent on healthy microbes in the soil to produce nitrates. With the presence of these nitrates, plants can absorb the minerals in the ground. The plants are dependent on the microbe population in the soil to grow. The microbe population is dependent on replenishing the soil with natural, mineral-rich compost. When the soil is not replenished with organic, mineral-rich compost, the microbe population quickly diminishes. At this point the plants do not produce crops, unless you add organic compost to feed a growing population of microbes.

When the soil is not replenished with organic, mineral-rich compost, the soil becomes mineral-deficient within ten years.

With modern fertilizer techniques, farmers learned to bypass the step of adding mineral-rich compost to the soil. Adding nitrates to the soil meant the plants could directly take the minerals that they needed to grow. The result is mineral-deficient produce and farmland that is dramatically mineral-deficient.

Ultimately, this problem will be solved with mineral supplementation to the land, along with organic gardening practices. Although you may be eating organic produce from the grocery store, it will still take many years before all the minerals are available to you. This problem can and will be solved one day, but not any time soon. In the meantime, you must supplement the food you eat with minerals.

During the last five years in my neighborhood, Marin County, California, we have suffered the tragic loss of thousands of oak trees. Thousands of trees are dying from what is being called sudden oak disease. We have three acres of dying oaks on our property, and my wife, Bonnie, has been trying to save them. With five years of experimentation and the help of many dedicated environmentalists, Bonnie has found a cure.

You guessed it—mineral supplementation. Adding mineral ash to the ground around the trees enables the oaks to fight off this scourge. Increasing the minerals in the soil doubles the microbe population every twenty-eight minutes. Within weeks, billions of new microbes are busy producing the nitrates necessary for the trees to assimilate the new minerals.

Increasing the minerals in the soil doubles the microbe population every twenty-eight minutes.

My wife has shared the solution with our California government representatives but has yet to receive a response. The state government has allotted $30 million to research this new problem. Perhaps such an inexpensive solution as spreading mineral ash seems too simple.

The growing awareness of mineral deficiency in the 1930s helped to popularize the health food industry. Even the government was exclaiming that everyone needed nutrient supplementation. A variety of mineral supplements and pills became available to the public. The movement lost its popularity because the mineral supplements didn't work. You cannot feed rocks to the body and expect the body to assimilate them.

You cannot feed rocks to the body and expect the body to assimilate them.

Even plants can't directly assimilate minerals. They require nitrates produced by microbes to stimulate the assimilation of minerals in the soil. Pills alone are not the answer. Since mineral supplements were not effective, the excitement about them waned.

Today there is a variety of natural plant source minerals that the body *can* assimilate. The best mineral supplements will have the words *plant source minerals, ionic plant source minerals,* or *colloidal plant source minerals* on the label. *Colloidal* and *ionic* mean that the minerals are so tiny that the cells can absorb them. In my experience, the ionic plant source minerals have the best effect. With the availability of these supplements, you can begin helping yourself and your children.

Within three days, ADD children once incapable of doing homework suddenly begin doing their homework. This kind of dramatic change is from minerals alone. When combined with all the elements of *The Mars and Venus Diet and Exercise Solution,* taking minerals is even more effective. Without successful mineral supplementation, all the other ingredients in this powerful mixture are incapable of producing the promised results.

Within three days, ADD children once incapable of doing homework suddenly begin doing their homework.

In some cases, people have written to me that the program was not working for them as it appears to work for others. Although no program can ever work the same for everyone, they were able to enjoy the many benefits of balanced brain chemistry by changing the brand of plant source minerals they were taking. The minerals make all the difference.

Although the understanding of the importance of trace minerals is new, researchers are discovering more about their importance each day. For example, the trace mineral boron is required for the body to assimilate the mineral calcium. We already know how important calcium is, but we didn't know that we also needed the trace mineral to assimilate our calcium supplies. If you are not getting enough boron in your diet, because the ground is deficient in it, then your body cannot assimilate the calcium in your food, drink, or supplements. In this manner, the importance of all seventy-seven minerals and trace minerals is gradually becoming recognized.

9

THE THREE EASY STEPS
OF THE MARS AND VENUS SOLUTION

The Mars and Venus Diet and Exercise Solution has three easy steps. By following each of these steps every day, you will quickly begin to produce the brain chemistry of health, happiness, and lasting romance. In this chapter, we will explore the three steps that are the core of the program.

STEP 1.
START YOUR DAY WITH WATER

Wake up each morning and drink 6 to 8 ounces of water and activate it with cleansing nutrients. As soon as you wake up and get out of bed, without thinking too much, prepare and then drink your activated water. To activate 8 ounces of water, add each of the following ingredients:

1. Juice from half a lemon
2. A teaspoon of honey or some juice for sweetness
3. A suggested portion of a high-quality ionic plant source trace mineral supplement
4. An ounce of aloe vera juice

Let's explore the importance of these four ingredients.

1. Lemon Power

When you think lemon, think Mr. Clean. Lemon and water are Mother Nature's most potent cleansers. Taken together, they are one of the oldest and most commonly used health remedies. Lemon and water can be found in almost all ancient traditions as an essential ingredient for good health and healing. Lemon juice and even its aroma is an antibacterial, antiseptic, and antiviral disinfectant that promotes white cell formation and improves immune function.

In the modern world, we commonly use lemon juice in our water to flavor it or in our dishwashing detergents because of its cleansing properties, but we don't regularly benefit from its healing abilities. If we wish to cleanse our bodies of toxins, the juice from half a lemon mixed with water is best used on an empty stomach upon awakening.

Lemon juice also has the effect of lowering high blood sugar. Whenever you can add lemon to a meal, it will assist you in sustaining healthy blood sugar levels. Adding lemon to a meal or dessert will slow down the release of sugar into the blood and lower high blood sugar by 30 percent.

Besides cleansing and helping to balance blood sugar, lemon juice also has the effect of making the body more alkaline. Most sickness is associated with too much acid in the cellular terrain of the body. Lemon in your water or your foods has the profound effect of normalizing the balance of acid and alkaline in the body.

Another product known to help make the body more alkaline is apple cider vinegar. It was popularized in the last century by the founder of the health food industry, Paul Bragg. Bragg Organic Apple Cider Vinegar is available in most health food grocery stores and can also be used to activate your cleansing drink.

2. A Spoonful of Sugar

A spoonful of sugar to help the medicine go down is not such a bad idea. It makes your morning drink taste better and feeds your brain as well. The brain gets all its energy from glucose, a sugar. When we eat sugar, the brain gets an immediate lift. That is why most people in our society tend to be addicted to sugar.

Sugar stimulates the production of dopamine and serotonin. It is the drug of choice for millions of people. It is not as harmful as street drugs, but it is just as addictive. Sugar does the same thing alcohol does for the alcoholic and cocaine does for the addict. It produces feel-good hormones in the brain. Sugar is a natural and healthy way to produce the brain chemistry of pleasure, motivation, clarity, happiness, and relaxation.

Refined sugar causes a momentary experience of healthy brain chemistry, but because the sugar is refined, the body is unable to sustain this production. Any carbohydrate breaks down gradually into sugar. Such complex carbohydrates as whole grains and vegetables provide a sustained release of glucose. Sugar feeds the brain, but eating refined sugar causes an instant rush. Once the body gets a taste of what it needs, it craves more. This gives rise to cravings for refined carbohydrates and sugar. We will explore later in Chapter 11 the many pitfalls of refined and processed sugars as well as potentially harmful sugar replacements.

Eating refined sugar inevitably reduces brain fuel.

Added to your morning drink, a little honey, fructose, or fruit juice gives the brain the energy it needs to get going. The brain needs oxygen and glucose to wake up and start doing what it is designed to do. Research demonstrates that increased sugar and oxygen enhance brain performance. In this healthy context, we can appreciate the wisdom of the adage "A spoonful of sugar makes the medicine go down."

3. Ionic Plant Source Trace Minerals

Trace minerals first thing in the morning are also essential to help the body begin its required cleansing process. If we were not so mineral-deficient already, the trace minerals in the lemon juice would be enough to activate all the cleansing processes in the body. The lemons grown today are also mineral-deficient. A lemon is not what it used to be.

By starting your day with all seventy-seven naturally occurring minerals and trace minerals, you will be getting the support your body needs not only to cleanse itself, but to begin producing the necessary chemicals and hormones in your brain. With this important beginning for the day, you will have the nutritional foundation to cope successfully with the inevitable stress you will encounter.

4. Aloe Vera Juice

Aloe vera is commonly used on the skin to heal sunburn. When taken internally, aloe vera juice also has a remarkable healing power for cleansing your body. Just as it soothes outer wounds, it relieves and heals our inner body. Toxic buildup results in the swelling of the body's tissues. Drinking aloe vera juice reduces internal swelling and strengthens the immune system in its battle against harmful bacteria, parasites, and viruses.

Drinking aloe vera juice reduces internal swelling
and strengthens the immune system.

The internal use of aloe vera is well documented. Major universities and research groups have published volumes of reports regarding the internal application of aloe vera. The studies are truly impressive.

You will find that aloe vera as a dietary supplement maintains normal, healthy stomach lining, digestion, and cell growth, and works as a general overall tonic. Aloe vera has attracted the attention of athletes and other highly active people interested in supporting and maintaining their overall energy levels.

Research has shown that aloe vera contains natural antibiotics, astringents, a pain inhibitor, and a growth stimulator to promote the healing of injured surfaces. Its healing properties have been recognized for centuries, by ancient Egyptians and Chinese as well as Alexander the Great. By delivering extra oxygen to the cells, aloe vera provides the body with the extra energy necessary to do its work.

By delivering extra oxygen to the cells, aloe vera provides the body with the extra energy necessary to do its work.

How can one little plant offer all these benefits? No one knows exactly how aloe vera accomplishes its amazing feats, but one major belief is that the gel of this plant rebuilds body tissue by stimulating the growth of cells. This may explain why there is little or no scar tissue after a burn or wound treated with aloe vera has healed. Aloe vera is hypoallergenic and has no known side effects, even when consumed in large amounts.

Aloe vera juice helps to detoxify the bowel, neutralize stomach acidity, and relieve constipation and gastric ulcers. It has the dramatic effect of balancing blood sugar. Patients with diabetes given aloe vera juice have experienced significant improvement.

Aloe vera reduces inflammation of the body's tissues, which is linked to all toxic conditions of the body, immune system disorders such as cancer and AIDS, and common food allergies. Its cleansing action not only helps the body remove toxins but also reduces the overgrowth of candida in the gut.

In general, drinking aloe vera juice each morning increases one's energy and well-being. By reducing inflammation, aloe vera allows the lymphatic system to do its cleansing job. With this support, the liver can in turn do its job of processing amino acids for the healthy production of hormones and brain chemicals.

Add one ounce of pure aloe vera juice to activate your water each morning. Make sure the brand you pick is cold processed and made from the whole leaf. Heat-processing of aloe vera kills all the important enzymes. Whole-leaf aloe vera has even more healing properties. Make sure that the aloe vera juice you purchase is not diluted. Some labels say pure aloe vera juice, but companies reduce the concentration to 10 percent aloe vera and 90 percent water. You want to get 100 percent aloe vera juice undiluted by water.

MAKING YOUR MORNING CLEANSING DRINK

By combining these four ingredients, you will be activating your morning water to assist your body to cleanse itself efficiently and to produce the necessary brain chemicals. You can mix all this together the night before in a bottle and then drink it immediately upon rising. You can make enough for the whole day to give you extra energy. Ideally, you should shake the whole mixture five to ten times in a shaker or bottle before drinking. Stirring it all together is good, but shaking is better. Shaking activates the potency of ionic trace minerals.

Ideally, you should shake the whole mixture five to ten times in a shaker or bottle before drinking.

Some health brands have minerals and aloe vera already in a drink. This miraculous activated drink is great in the morning, but it can also be used throughout the day. It will give you an extra lift beyond drinking just plain water. During the day, you can drink up to an ounce for every 8 ounces of water.

STEP 2.
BOUNCE, SHAKE, BREATHE, AND FLEX—
THE EXERCISE PORTION

The second step of *The Mars and Venus Diet and Exercise Solution* is to bounce, shake, breathe, and flex. When you exercise, you will always begin and end with the bounce and shake exercise. In between, you will perform your favorite exercises. To create healthy brain chemistry, you should choose exercises that are easy to perform. The philosophy of "No pain, no gain" doesn't apply to the Mars and Venus Solution. When exercise routines require too much metabolic activity, they interfere with the brain's ability to create a balanced brain chemistry.

Intense exercise can interfere with the brain's ability to create a balanced brain chemistry.

With intense exercise, the blood sugar levels necessary for brain functioning may drop too much, and important amino acids necessary to create brain chemistry and hormones are directed to the muscles instead of to the brain and other glands. The increased metabolic activity of intense exercise or prolonged jogging requires the burning of additional minerals. These minerals are often leached right out of the bones, resulting in mineral deficiency and premature aging, not to mention osteoporosis.

Intense exercise is necessary to build muscles. In moderation, it is good for you, but too much becomes an obstacle to good health. You may look good, but your body and relationships will suffer. If you are primarily interested in managing weight, toning your muscles, and creating healthy brain chemistry, intense exercise is not necessary. If you are overweight, it is better to avoid intense exercise until you get back to your healthy weight. Then you can easily gauge the right amount for you.

> If you are overweight, it is better to avoid intense exercise until you get back to your healthy weight.

People born with more muscular bodies have a greater need for intense exercise. Although it is not a necessity for health, weight, and stress management, intense exercise is an important pleasure in life. If intense workouts are fun, then they are generally healthy. If they are much longer than forty minutes, they are probably accelerating the aging process.

More and more evidence is pointing out the common symptoms of overexercising. Although a reduction in performance is normally considered a sign of overtraining, it can be *preceded* by changes in mood. The overtraining syndrome for someone following an anaerobic training program such as strength training manifests itself as anxiety or agitation. In contrast, an overtrained state caused by aerobic exercise can lead to feelings of depression.

> With intense exercise you may look good, but your health and relationships will suffer.

For obese men, additional intense weight-bearing exercise is very helpful to increase muscle mass and burn fat. It is easier for men to burn fat by exercising because they have more muscle mass from birth. By building his muscle mass, an obese man dramatically increases his metabolism and can burn fat more efficiently.

Obese women need to avoid intense exercise. Moderate exercise is all they need. Intense exercise encourages fat-burning mitochondrial cells in women to burn carbohydrates and not fats. While sweating and struggling with intense exercise routines, obese women are mistakenly inhibiting their body's ability to burn fat. The benefit of intense exercise for men is that it activates the metabolism to burn fat throughout the day. Intense exercise does not affect women so favorably. Research studies reveal that women who do regular, moderately intense exercise burn more fat than they would with more intense exercise programs.

Obese women need to avoid intense exercise.

The bounce and shake exercise, accompanied by some easy stretches from beginner's yoga, Pilates, tai chi, chi kung, the Five Rites, or Callanetics, are all you need to activate your metabolism and stimulate brain chemistry.

The Bounce and Shake Technique

Immediately after drinking your activated water, begin the bounce and shake technique and continue it for one to three minutes. If you want to burn fat for weight management, bounce and shake for up to five minutes.

This technique is the most effective fat-burning technique. It not only activates the lymphatic system for cleansing but also stimulates the flow of energy in the body. When you stop the technique after a few minutes, you can feel energy tingling throughout your body while you stand still.

This tingling results from the cells in your body vibrating faster. This vibration generates cellular electricity, which can be conducted throughout the body by adequate levels of water, oxygen, and minerals. This energy is call *chi* energy by the Chinese and *prana* by the Indians. A version of the bounce and shake routine is present in most of the world's oldest healing traditions.

When done after drinking activated water and on an empty stomach, this simple movement will dramatically increase your metabolism so that you will be burning more calories all day. Even when you are sitting in front of a computer monitor or riding in your car, your revved-up metabolism will continue burning fat reserves most efficiently.

The bounce and shake technique increases your metabolism so that you will be burning more calories all day.

You don't need to take a long time and exert a lot of energy to burn calories through a rigorous exercise routine; Step 2 of *The Mars and Venus Diet and Exercise Solution* will focus on easy-to-perform exercises that primarily activate your metabolism to continue burning calories at a higher rate throughout the day and night.

The bounce and shake exercise provides benefits in these four ways:

1. The increased cellular vibration burns fat, tones your muscles, and increases your lean body mass.

2. While bouncing and shaking, you will also flex your spine in coordination with deeper-than-usual breathing. The rhythmic flexing of the spine increases vitality and stimulates the healthy production of brain chemistry by pumping spinal fluid into and out of the brain.

3. The increased oxygen from rhythmic breathing will also stimulate your metabolism to burn fat more efficiently during the day.

4. The gentle whole-body movement of bounce and shake stimulates the lymphatic system to purify and cleanse the body.

Let's now break down the six steps of the bounce and shake technique.

1. Standing with knees slightly bent, feet comfortably apart, bounce up and down easily without lifting your heels off the ground.

2. As you bounce, let your arms hang in a relaxed and floppy

manner by your side. Shake your hands by your side as you bounce up and down.

3. While you gently bounce and shake, slowly nod your head up and down in a comfortable range of no more than two to four inches.

4. As you nod back and look up, breathe in through your nose to the count of five seconds, and then exhale to the count of five seconds as you lower your head.

5. During the first minute, breathe in and out through your nose. During the next minute, breathe in and out through your nose while making a noise originating at the base of your throat. This sound comes from the air flowing through your throat and not your vocal chords. You will sound like you are quietly snoring. During the remaining one to three minutes, breathe in through your nose and out through your mouth. When you exhale through your mouth, pucker your lips and blow out as if you were trying to put out a candle two feet in front of you.

6. Stop bouncing and shaking. While standing in a relaxed position, take a quiet minute simply to feel the tingling in your body. This is best felt while standing straight with arms relaxed by your side and knees slightly bent. Besides the important aspect of activating your lymphatic system, this vibration is the activation of billions of cells to make you healthy.

Of all the exercises I practice, bounce and shake is the most important. Being sedentary puts our lymphatic system to sleep, and the burden of cleansing the body is put on the liver. When you feel overwhelmed or tired in life, that is precisely what your liver is feeling. If the lymphatic system is not working effectively, then your liver is overworked. The liver can't do its job of transforming digested proteins into neurotransmitters if it is toxic and overworked. This program provides the foundation for your body to create the brain chemistry of health, happiness, and romance. Any kind of aerobic exercise stimulates the lymphatic system, but not nearly as much as the simple technique of bounce and shake.

> The liver can't do its job of transforming
> digested proteins into neurotransmitters
> if it is toxic and overworked.

Breathe and Flex Your Spine

After you have completed the bounce and shake exercise, you are ready to do about ten to twenty minutes of gentle exercise. Most low-intensity exercise or stretch routines will assist you in breathing more deeply while gently flexing your spine to begin pumping and circulating brain chemicals in and out of the brain. For healthy brain chemistry, the cerebral spinal fluid needs to flow freely to and from the brain. Sitting in chairs and cars restricts the flow of cerebral spinal fluid. By taking time to flex the spine in the morning, you give your brain the help it needs to create healthy brain chemistry. When you flex your spine, the cerebral spinal fluid flows freely like a pure and clean river instead of stagnating like a murky pond.

Many popular stretching and exercise programs are sufficient to stimulate healthy brain chemistry when they are also associated with sustained and relaxed breathing. Oxygen is the most important nutrient for the brain. Twenty percent of the oxygen we breathe is required by the brain. The human brain weighs about three pounds, less than 2 percent of our body weight, and yet requires 20 percent of our oxygen supply to function. By increasing your oxygen supply, your brain will get what it needs to be healthy.

> Oxygen is the most important nutrient
> for the brain.

When you exercise, make sure to sustain a constant breath in and out to the count of five seconds without ever getting out of breath. Use each of these three types of breathing: head, chest, and abdomen.

1. **Head breathing** requires inhaling and exhaling through the nose with an emphasis on filling your head and nasal passages full of air. With each inhale, slightly lift your head up as if to look at the ceiling, and on the exhale let your head come back down as if you are looking a little below the horizon. This range of movement is very slight—between two and four inches. During gentle stretching exercises, breathe using this head breathing technique to the count of five in and five out.

2. **Chest breathing** requires breathing in and out the nose, with emphasis on filling your lungs while expanding your rib cage to the sides. During chest breathing, also make a slight sound or tone from the base of the throat as the breath flows in and out. This tone sounds like a quiet snore. Throughout the whole series of chest breathing exercises, keep the volume of air the same. During moderate exercise breath, use chest breathing to the count of five in and five out.

3. **Abdomen breathing** for moderately intense exercise. Breathe in through your nose, pucker your lips, and blow out your mouth on the exhale. This more intense breathing is used in many hospitals to help patients assimilate more oxygen in the cells. It is commonly taught to patients who have chronic obstructive pulmonary disease or to those who become short of breath with minimal exertion. Hospitals call it pursed lip breathing (so the insurance will pay for sessions!).

The action of exhaling with pursed lips actually creates a little back pressure in the lungs that facilitates expansion of the alveoli and better oxygen exchange. The alveoli are small sacs in your lungs that hold the air you breathe. Miraculously, patients' oxygen saturations go up dramatically after doing pursed lip breathing for a minute or two.

Each of these three kinds of breathing is effective, but what is important is a consistent rhythm. When considering the production of brain chemistry, consistent breathing is the most important part of any exercise routine. Any of the following suggested exercise routines will stimulate the production of brain chemicals when accompanied with five-second breathing:

- Do any easy-to-perform basic exercise or stretching routine such as yoga, Pilates, tai chi, chi kung, the Five Rites, or Callanetics. The best routine for you is one that motivates you to keep doing it. For your exercise to be most effective in producing brain chemicals, you must never get out of breath or feel sore afterwards.
- Go for a walk or easy jog, but make sure not to get out of breath. Sustain a breath count of five seconds in and five seconds out at all times. Generally speaking, twenty minutes of aerobic exercise is all anyone needs. Unless you are in perfect shape, any more is often too much and wears out your body, triggering premature aging.
- If you are seeking to build muscle, then do that after twenty minutes of *easy* exercise. Give your brain a chance to produce the chemistry it requires first, and follow the thirty-minute program with a more strenuous weight training routine.
- When you do intense exercise, try to sustain the five-second easy breathing cycle and be careful not to overexercise to the point of sore muscles. If your muscles are sore afterwards or the next day, you may be building muscles, but you are not stimulating the production of brain chemicals.
- With brief moments of intensity, you can build muscles without injuring them or feeling sore afterwards. Overexercise is not necessary to build muscles. Sore muscles are a sign that most of your amino acids are being directed to the muscles for repair. They are then not available to be used by your brain. This explains the brain fog athletes often experience.
- When working out at the gym, as long as you don't overexercise and you maintain regular five-second in and out

breathing, you will get the benefits of healthy brain chemistry and body building both.

Most important in picking the best exercise routine for you is to pick a routine you enjoy. Research shows that most people only stick with regular exercise for six months and then quit. Unless you stay motivated, your exercise routine is of little value because you will stop it after a while.

**Your exercise routine is of little value
if you don't do it.**

Finish Up with Bounce and Shake

After your ten to twenty minutes of exercise, drink another 6- to 8-ounce glass of activated water and do the bounce and shake technique again. This time make a small adjustment. Instead of shaking your hands back and forth in a relaxed fashion, firmly extend your fingers toward the floor (like karate chops) and vigorously shake your hands downward by the side of your body. When you are finished, take another minute to stand in a relaxed position, with head level and chest up, feeling your body tingling.

If it is difficult to think of devoting twenty to thirty minutes every day to exercise when you get up, start out with just five minutes of bounce and shake. As you continue for a week, you will start waking up earlier and have extra time to exercise.

Following this routine for a few weeks will activate your metabolism. Not only will you have more energy and normalize your weight, but your sleep patterns will change as well. When your body and metabolism are normal, it becomes easy to wake up a little earlier so you can do a half hour of exercise. With an active metabolism during the day and balanced amounts of brain chemistry, you will be able to go to sleep a little earlier and sleep much more soundly.

With a more active metabolism, you create more time by needing less sleep.

After twenty to thirty minutes of exercise, complete your normal bathroom routine. When you are ready for breakfast, it is time for the third step of the Mars and Venus Solution.

STEP 3.
DRINK YOUR BREAKFAST SHAKE

The third step is to prepare and drink your Mars and Venus nutrient-dense breakfast shake. By blending together all the necessary ingredients for creating healthy brain chemistry, you will replace your usual breakfast with something much more nutritious. This healthy shake can replace breakfast or it can supplement a light and healthy breakfast. (In Chapter 11, we explore the ingredients of a healthy meal.) If you are overweight, just have the shake every day until you have achieved your ideal weight. By combining the right elements, you will get everything your body needs and you will feel satisfied. This is not a deprivation diet plan.

A diet does not have to mean deprivation.

If you are overweight, you don't need to eat so much for breakfast. A low-calorie nutrient-dense breakfast will burn your extra fat to get energy. The more overweight you are, the fewer calories you will require in your breakfast shake. All that extra fat consists of calories waiting to be burned. We have already discussed that a low-calorie nutrient-dense breakfast signals your body to burn the extra fuel. On the other hand, eating a *high*-calorie breakfast will tell your body that you don't need to use your extra fat. As a result, your metabolism slows down. Eating a low-calorie breakfast is very different from skipping breakfast altogether.

A high-calorie breakfast will tell your body
to slow down the metabolism and hold on
to extra fat.

Skipping breakfast will turn down your metabolism and inhibit the burning of fat. When you skip breakfast, your body turns down the metabolism to store energy. If there is no food around, it decides to conserve what it's got.

This doesn't necessarily mean that you will not have energy in the morning, but it will set the pace for running out of steam as the day wears on. Without the dopamine stimulation of work or a new and exciting relationship, men become exhausted when they get home. Without the serotonin stimulation of a nurturing relationship at the end of the day or the nurturing support of relaxed communication with friends during the day, many women feel increasingly overwhelmed.

By skipping breakfast, we run out of brain
chemicals by the end of the day.

The most important element of the Mars and Venus Solution is to drink a breakfast shake every day. When you have a low-calorie nutrient-dense breakfast shake, your body is bathed in an abundance of nutrients, so your metabolism doesn't slow down. Because your meal is low in calories, your body begins to burn extra fat.

Understanding fat burning is like basic economics. If you are out of work, you stop spending and hold on to what you've got. If you miss breakfast, your metabolism slows down to avoid burning all the energy. On the other hand, if you have a great job with regular cash flow but are a little low in your checking account, you draw from your savings account. By eating a low-calorie, nutrient-rich breakfast (a good job with regular cash flow), your body begins converting stored fat to burn for extra energy (you pull some money from your savings account).

If you are overweight, 200 to 300 calories of a nutrient-dense breakfast shake will be the perfect amount. If that doesn't seem enough, promise yourself another shake in a couple of hours or a tasty treat later. By starting the day in this way, you can then go on to having a snack a few hours later, a much bigger lunch, another snack in the afternoon, and a moderate-size dinner. If you skip breakfast or don't have a big enough lunch, you will want to eat too many calories for dinner. Having a low-calorie but nutrient-rich breakfast will stimulate fat burning and will feed your cells so that you are not always wanting to eat more and more.

The more overweight you are, the fewer calories you will require for breakfast.

As you regain your normal weight, you can add a little more of each ingredient, making the shake now more than 500 calories, or you can use the low-calorie shake. If you choose to eat regular breakfast foods, make sure to complement your breakfast with at least 200 calories of nutritional supplementation in a shake. Whether you are underweight or overweight, when you achieve your ideal weight, you don't need more than 500 calories for breakfast.

If you wish to follow government recommendations, which I believe are still a little too high in calories, then have 500 calories for breakfast, a lunch of 500 to 1,000 calories, two snacks of 250 calories each, and 500 calories for dinner. This will give you the recommended 2,000 to 2,500 calories a day. Keep in mind that as you get older, you are maintaining your body, not building it. Unless you are on a body-building program, you don't need so many calories.

As you get older, you are only maintaining your body, and thus your body requires fewer calories.

These figures are for those who really want to count calories. *The Mars and Venus Diet and Exercise Solution* suggests that you eat a low-calorie breakfast and open your mind to eating fewer calories during the day. Do your best to eat healthy food whenever possible, and eat as much as you want. When you have a healthy breakfast, unless you go out of balance with some junk food, your body will hunger for the right amount of food for you.

While seeking out healthy foods, don't become so regimented that you feel deprived. Feeling deprived will always lead to unhealthy cravings later and to psychological imbalance.

It is generally better to eat junk food than no food at all. Even junk food is not so bad if you supplement it with a few enzyme and mineral capsules. Since most foods we eat today are nutrient-deficient, it's a good idea to supplement even a healthy meal with enzymes and minerals. If you don't have your mineral and enzyme supplements, try to start the meal with a salad and take a little longer to chew it. This will stimulate the production of enzymes to digest your meal.

**It is generally better to eat junk food
than to skip a meal.**

Never miss a meal and don't deprive yourself if possible. As you begin producing the dopamine and serotonin your brain needs, your tastes will change, your diet will become healthier, and you will naturally want to eat healthier foods in the right amount for you.

With this program, you will have so much energy that you won't need coffee, refined-sugar desserts and drinks, and other stimulants. Your morning shake will give you much more energy than tea or coffee does. Your stress levels will normalize, and you will not need to drink alcohol to relax or to enjoy your evening.

This doesn't mean that you can't ever enjoy black tea, coffee, desserts, and alcohol as occasional treats. Although these substances have negative effects on your body, they often have good effects on your mind and heart. Coffee or black tea is for some an emotional anchor associated with the comfort of spending time with good friends. Likewise, drinking alcohol may bring up feelings linked to friendship, fun, and ease. With the healthy influence of a nutrient-dense diet and the production of healthy brain chemistry, most people can handle a moderate amount of these unhealthy treats.

Junk food may be toxic to the body, but it also has sentimental value for the mind and heart.

Anything unhealthy that you have to do every day is clearly a serious addiction. *The Mars and Venus Diet and Exercise Solution* frees you from your addictions to unhealthy substances so that you don't have to ingest them every day. Without cravings for unhealthy food, you are free to make better choices. In moderation, these emotional indulgences are okay if you are healthy. To heal a sick body, an overweight body, or an underweight body, you must avoid junk foods for a while. This task becomes much easier when you are producing adequate brain chemicals.

To heal a sick body, you must avoid toxic foods until you get well.

Without the dehydrating effects of coffee, your body can more effectively absorb nutrients and minerals to cleanse and heal itself. Without the toxic load associated with drinking alcohol, your liver can begin to heal itself. Without the leaching of minerals from your bones associated with eating refined sugars, your cells and bones can begin to heal themselves. With the abundance of minerals made available in your morning wake-up routine and breakfast shake, you have provided your body with everything it needs to create healthy brain chemistry.

If you feed your cells and brain in the morning, your tastes automatically begin to change in about nine days; healthful foods actually start to taste better. In the beginning, to assist your body in letting go of old, unhealthy habits, try to surround yourself with healthier foods and avoid looking at junk food or having access to it.

Just seeing junk food can trigger an emotional hunger, even though your body doesn't really want it or need anything at that moment. Eating junk food in the past was generally associated with a deficiency of brain chemistry and a mood imbalance. Just looking at junk food reminds your body of those times. This can trigger an imbalance, which activates an addictive hunger or craving.

Until the trauma of a lifetime of junk food is healed, avoid exposure to it. This is similar to psychological healing. If someone has hurt you, you would not put his or her picture up in your bedroom to look at before you go to bed or when you wake up to heal the hurt.

How Much to Eat

When your cells are getting fed in the morning, you will begin eating more healthy quantities of food. Say good-bye to calorie counting and deprivation diets. In this program, you have to eat at least three meals and try to get in two snacks as well. Eat as much as your body wants. In the beginning, use a little restraint if you know you are eating too much. Soon it will take no willpower; you will want to eat only the amount of food your body needs and can digest.

Ideally, breakfast and dinner should be our lower-calorie meals and lunch our biggest meal. The body starts producing enzymes to digest our food around 7 A.M. Between 7 A.M. and noon, enzyme production increases to a maximum. From 2 P.M., enzyme production starts to decline, and at 7 P.M., production stops. If you eat after 7 P.M., you need to supplement your meals with plant source digestive enzymes. Since most of our food is cooked or processed, it is a good idea to supplement every meal with plant source minerals and enzymes.

The Ingredients of the Mars and Venus Shake

I will provide you with a list of the suggested ingredients for your Mars and Venus shake with the precise amounts for each ingredient. The closer you get to these amounts, the more effective the program will be. Since everyone is different, you certainly need to give yourself the latitude to develop your own perfect breakfast routine. Remember, these ingredients are simply healthful foods. There are no dangerous side effects from eating food substances in moderation. If, however, you are diabetic and are giving yourself insulin shots, you must be careful to monitor your blood sugar levels. As your body begins to produce healthier insulin levels on its own, it would be unhealthy to increase insulin levels with a shot.

Low Calorie

You can blend your own breakfast shake with 200 to 400 calories of good and wholesome natural food supplements. All health food supplements list the amounts of protein, fat, and carbohydrates they contain in grams. To determine the number of fat, protein, and carbohydrate calories, multiply fat grams by 9, protein grams by 4, and carbohydrate grams by 4.

  1. **Carbohydrates.** Total carbohydrate calories should be 50 percent, or 25 to 50 grams (one gram of carbohydrate is generally equal to 4 calories). If your exercise routine includes intense weight training, even more carbohydrates are required. By adding a banana, you gain another 100 calories. Try to avoid packaged shakes that contain refined sugars. High quality fructose- or fruit-sweetened products are much better than sugar, dextrose, sucrose, malt syrup, corn syrup, high fructose, or any of the sugar-free sweeteners that have aspartame or the new chemical additive sucralose, which is sold in many "low-carb" products under the name Splenda. You can add fresh or

frozen fruit to supply your carbohydrate balance. Here is a list of fruits and how many calories they contain:

Fruit	Portion	Calories
Apple juice	4 fl oz	58
Carrot juice	4 fl oz	50
Cranberry juice	4 fl oz	73
Grape juice	4 fl oz	78
Orange juice	4 fl oz	55
Papaya nectar	4 fl oz	71
Pear nectar	4 fl oz	73
Pineapple juice	4 fl oz	68
Apple	1 med	81
Apricot	3	51
Banana	1 med	100
Blackberries	1 cup	72
Cantaloupe	1 cup	57
Dates	2	44
Figs	1 med	37
Grapes	1 cup	58
Orange	1 med	65
Papaya	1 med	58
Peach	1 med	37
Pear	1 med	98
Pineapple	1 cup	77
Pineapple, canned	1 cup	200
Raisins	1 cup	450
Raspberries	1 cup	61
Strawberries	1 cup	45
Strawberries, frozen and sweetened	1 cup	245
Watermelon	1 cup	50

Referring to this chart, you can easily determine how much carbohydrate sweetening you will need in your morning Mars and Venus shake. For an extra boost of brain chemistry, add cassava powder and/or maca powder. Both of these imported starches (which are similar to potatoes) have special benefits. Cassava, also called yucca, is widely used in tropical countries and is commonly associated with tapioca. It is one of the highest serotonin-producing foods. It is great for both men and women. Maca, another amazing import, comes from Peru. It is an energizing food without caffeine that increases stamina and mental clarity and other symptoms of dopamine. With this in your shake, you will never need coffee again. Maca is also a powerful aphrodisiac for both men and women.

2. Protein powder. Find a high quality protein powder product to put in your blend. Protein should be at least 30 percent of the total calories for men and 20 percent of the total calories for women. Too much protein for women may inhibit the production of serotonin. Not enough protein for men will inhibit the production of dopamine in the brain.

Men generally need about 13 to 30 grams of protein; 23 is an average amount. If you are more muscular and weigh 200 or more pounds and you are not overweight, you can probably use 30 grams. If you get sleepy, then it was too much. Women generally need about 10 to 20 grams of protein.

The benefit of using a protein powder is that you can make sure you are getting all the essential amino acids while controlling the fat and carbohydrate content of the meal. Blended shakes give you a rich source of all the nutrients you would want in a meal, without the extra calories.

3. Grind and add flaxseeds for essential omega-3 fatty acids. Put in at least 20 percent good fats for men and 30 percent good fats for women. While this percentage of fat may seem high for some, it is not high when we are considering 30 percent of 200 to 400 calories. The best way to give your body good fats is to use a high-speed blender and add a couple of tablespoons of flaxseeds for women and about one tablespoon for men. By grinding flaxseeds, you will get high quality omega-3 essential fatty acids. One tablespoon of flaxseeds is 15 grams and contains 5.7 grams of fat.

You can also add hemp seeds. Hemp seeds are *not* marijuana, and they can be ordered online from Canadian sources. They don't need much grinding at all. Another effective approach is to add flaxseed oil. One tablespoon is about 13 grams of fat, which is plenty for women. Men need a little more than half a tablespoon to get the 8 grams they generally require.

If you get a little foggy in the brain or sleepy, then you have taken too much good fat. For variety in taste, you can also add a handful of walnuts to get omega-3 fatty acids.

If you are not grinding flaxseeds for your dietary fast, then it is also a good idea to buy some flax meal and have a couple of tablespoons. Flax meal contains omega-3 oil, and it provides a lot of good fiber.

4. Enzymes. Add high quality full spectrum plant source enzymes from your health food store. Make sure there is a full range of different digestive enzymes.

5. Vitamins. Add a high quality multivitamin. Make sure it has a full range of B vitamins. B vitamins, along with vitamin C and folic acid, are required to transform amino acids into the neurotransmitters dopamine and serotonin. To eliminate cravings for refined sugar, look for a chromium supplement with 150 micrograms a day or 25 to 50 micrograms a meal as well.

6. Ionic plant source trace minerals. Most important, add a generous portion of plant source trace minerals and calcium/magnesium supplements. If your mineral supplement doesn't easily dissolve in water, it probably will not dissolve or be assimilated in your body. As we have already discussed, high quality minerals are the most important part of this program.

7. Water and ice. Add five or six cubes of ice and 6 to 8 ounces of water and then blend your shake. If you use juice instead of water, take into consideration that juice is to be counted as a carbohydrate. Ice makes the whole mixture taste better. If you are trying to lose weight, it will help activate your metabolism.

In the Ayurvedic tradition in India, people are discouraged from eating ice. This is appropriate for people who have very active lives just trying to survive, and thus active metabolisms. They also lived in a time when minerals were abundant in the diet.

The reason ice is good for losing weight is that it stimulates the body to heat up. When ice is ingested, the body has to compensate and heat back up to maintain a healthy and consistent body temperature, burning calories. In India, where it is hot, eating ice would overheat the body. They did not have the luxury of air conditioning on hot days.

When healthy people devote two hours to exercise, which dramatically raises the metabolism, it is appropriate to swear off ice, because they don't want to overheat the body. If you are overheated from exercise, ingesting ice is not a good thing. For those who do not exercise two or more hours, ice and cold refreshing water is fine. The water in the mountain streams of the Himalayas is always cold, and Indian yogis drink it cold and thrive.

When you have finished your blended shake, drink another glass of cool water to help your body assimilate the blended shake.

These seven ingredients may seem like a lot, but once you have all of them, it takes only a couple of minutes to prepare. You will not only have more time in the morning, but you will have more energy throughout the day. With this blend, you will begin to enjoy all the benefits of creating the brain chemistry of health, happiness, and lasting romance.

If during the day you experience hunger, have a little snack or make another blend with these seven ingredients. Keep in mind that every time you prepare a shake, you must drink it within fifteen minutes. You cannot put it in a thermos to take for a snack or meal replacement later. Once you blend the proteins and enzymes with water, the enzymes become active, digesting the proteins.

Every time you prepare a shake, you must drink it within fifteen minutes.

This process of digestion needs to take place in your stomach and not in a thermos. Predigested proteins will not taste good, nor will they have the same healthy effect on your body. It is similar to leaving food out too long. It begins to decompose, smell awful, and then eventually go bad.

You can't take a blended shake with you, but you can bring the mix. When I travel, I bring the ingredients along and make a shake in a couple of minutes. When I am too busy for a meal, I make a shake instead of missing the meal completely.

You can also go to the health food store and buy all seven ingredients, or you can use one of many reputable brands that already provide many of these ingredients in one package. As I mentioned in Chapter 2, I use the Isagenix brand, which is available at www.roadtohealth.Isagenix.com or customer service at 1-877-877-8111. Other brands available at your health store or at General Nutrition Centers are usually high in quality.

ACCELERATED WEIGHT MANAGEMENT

Weight management includes losing extra fat, gaining more lean muscle mass, and stabilizing ideal body fat levels and weight. All three can be accomplished with *The Mars and Venus Diet and Exercise Solution*. If you are underweight, you can begin to gain weight by building your muscle mass. If you are overweight, you can begin burning excess fat to lose that extra weight. Once you get to your ideal weight, the same program helps you to maintain your ideal weight without having to deprive yourself in any way.

Since so many people are overweight, we will first focus on burning extra fat to lose weight, then on maintaining your ideal weight, and finally, on building lean muscle mass and gaining weight if necessary. Losing weight through increased fat burning is accomplished by combining four important ingredients:

1. Cleansing
2. Activating your metabolism
3. A diet low in calories but high in nutrition
4. Eating to produce balanced brain chemistry

The Mars and Venus Solution does all this, and as a result, your body will begin to burn fat more effectively and much faster than with most popular effective weight loss programs. You can lose two or three pounds a week. With a cleaner liver and a normal metabolism, you will lose about 10 pounds in four weeks. In two months, the extra 20 pounds you may be carrying around right now will be gone. By continuing to follow the program, you will easily keep this weight off.

If you wish to lose weight faster, you can accelerate this process in a safe but effective manner without the use of harmful diet pills that contain ephedra or ephedrine, ma-huang, Fen-Phen, or caffeine. These substances speed up your metabolism by putting a strain on your heart and have been shown to be unhealthy. By giving your body a greater opportunity to cleanse itself automatically, you will begin to lose weight much faster.

**Diet pills to speed up your metabolism
are not healthy.**

Obesity is a sickness and your body is already designed to heal it like any sickness. All your body needs is a little help from you. To activate your body's self-healing ability to burn fat, you have to first give your liver a break from having to process the toxins you eat. From years of overeating, your body is filled with toxins that are being stored in excess fat. If you focus on cleansing your body by observing a two-day fast from eating solid foods, your liver gets a break from having to process new foods and can begin to process and cleanse the body of stored toxins.

Generally speaking, when you miss meals, it will inhibit fat burning. When you miss a meal or two, you give your body the message that there is not enough food. Your metabolism drops, and fat burning is inhibited. Fasting from solid foods is different from missing a meal. You may be missing a few meals, but you are still giving your body many of the nutrients that it needs. If you drink lots of nutrient-rich activated water, along with lots of stretching and breathing exercises, your body will take this opportunity to cleanse itself.

Rather than burn fat for energy, your body begins to burn fat to cleanse. This cleansing process gets activated when you replace your meals with water, lemon, minerals, aloe vera, and a little fruit sugar or honey. With these ingredients, your liver gets the green light to begin cleansing the body of old toxins. Fasting with lemon and honey is one of the oldest healing remedies in the world. It has been an integral part of every healing and spiritual tradition in the world.

Fasting with lots of water and low-intensity exercise activates accelerated fat burning to release body toxins.

A two-day fast will dramatically accelerate the process of losing weight. It works so much better than simply dieting, because it is not based on burning fat for energy. Research has shown that eating a low-calorie diet and getting plenty of exercise will burn only 1½ pounds of fat a week. When you are fasting and successfully cleansing the body, you can easily lose half a pound to a pound of weight a day.

If you fast instead of just diet, your body can burn a pound of fat a day.

Men may tend to lose a little more and women will tend to lose a little less than a pound a day. That's right—a pound a day. This is five times faster than long-term deprivation diets and intense exercise. Let's look at two of the thousands who have benefited from this cleansing program.

Jim was able to lose 31 pounds in thirty-three days. For Jim, it was all off his waist. Even better, he was able to keep it off. In thirty days, Jim lost a full seven inches from his waist. He started out at 205 pounds, and thirty-three days later, he weighed 174. On the maintenance diet, he continued to lose weight until he had achieved his ideal weight of 165 pounds.

At sixty-seven years of age, Jim realized that his weight had gradually increased and his body was getting out of control! The thought of dieting was not very appealing, although he knew something had to go. When he heard about this cleansing program, he thought he could tolerate nine days of suffering for this good cause. Like most people who follow this plan, he was delighted to discover there was no suffering! He felt energized, not hungry, not nervous or jittery, and not sleepy at all. In fact, he felt great—very alert and sharp.

The real thrill came when he measured and weighed himself— 31 pounds in thirty-three days, and seven inches off his waist! Imagine the excitement he felt when his tuxedo—made to measure twenty years ago—was once again a perfect fit!

I know that excitement, because using this program I was able to lose fifteen pounds in eighteen days, and suddenly all my clothes started to fit again. I was able to fit into the tuxedo from my wedding eighteen years ago.

Marge is a nutrition consultant and has been recommending nutritional programs to her clients for more than twenty years. She is always searching for new ideas and products to help her clients succeed. After seeing the amazing weight loss results in her good friend Peter, she was inspired and decided to test the nine-day cleansing program.

After one nine-day cycle, she had lost 21 inches and 13.5 pounds! Everyone started to notice as her face was changing along with her waistline. For the next thirty days, she took a morning mineral and aloe vera drink with a low-calorie nutritional shake for breakfast. She followed this with a low-calorie lunch and dinner, with two extra snacks at midmorning and midafternoon. With balanced brain chemistry from her morning cleanse and shake, she could easily eat 1,500 calories a day without feeling hungry. After this thirty-day cycle, she lost another 12.5 pounds and 15 more inches. It was such a thrill for her to see her true self appear after years of diet struggles. In thirty-seven days, she lost a total of 26 pounds and 36 inches.

Like so many thousands of people who have experienced this program, Marge was able to lose pounds and inches very quickly. After these thirty days, she shared, "I feel so alive and energetic. I have no carbohydrate cravings and have eliminated mood swings. My body feels totally balanced and I sleep fewer hours, more soundly—and without night sweats. I am so excited to have something this healthy as part of my life . . . and that I can offer my clients a better way. I am just thrilled. I feel wonderful as well as look great." Each day she continues to use the cleansing drink in the morning and replace breakfast with a nutritious morning shake.

NINE DAYS AND NINE POUNDS

How did Jim and Marge do it? They followed this simple three-step cleansing program.

1. **Two-day fast.** For the first two days, do a cleansing fast.

2. **Five-day, low-calorie diet.** For the next five days, eat a low-calorie, highly nutritious diet. For these five days, replace your breakfast and dinner with a low-calorie (about 250 calories) meal-replacement shake with all the ingredients of the Mars and Venus Solution. For lunch, have a regular healthy meal, avoiding processed breads, refined sugars, and dairy products.

3. **Two-day fast.** Finish this nine-day cycle with another two-

day cleansing fast. These last two days will stabilize the results of the first seven days. Every time you feel better and brighter, your body wants to cleanse itself to sustain this healthier state. After the first seven days, you will feel so much better that your body will begin to purify again. This last two-day cleanse is essential to stabilize the benefits of the program. After nine days, you will lose an average of a pound a day. Many women lose fewer pounds but more in inches. Many men lose an average of 15 pounds in nine days.

In Jim's case, he lost 15 pounds in his first nine-day cycle. After waiting a few weeks, he started another nine-day cycle and lost 16 pounds. In thirty-three days, he lost 31 pounds. You can do just one cycle or several to accelerate your gradual weight loss. Jim chose two. Some people have lost more than 60 pounds in a few months by repeating the nine-day cycle again and again over several months while enjoying the benefits of increasing health and vitality.

Thousands of people have already used this simple cleansing program to lose and keep off a pound a day. At my weekend workshops, we will begin this program together with the two-day fast. After just two days, many women would lose two dress sizes.

Enjoying a fun seminar, attendees were able to fill themselves with love instead of food, expel toxins, and miraculously heal symptoms of hypertension, diabetes, obesity, arthritis, skin diseases, insomnia, migraine headaches, and other chronic ailments in just a few days. Everyone feels so much better after a fast. Doing a fast with others and doing exercises throughout the day makes it much easier.

Everyone always feels better
and sleeps better after a fast.

At home alone, fasting can be more challenging, but if you are motivated, then it is easy. As toxins are released into the bloodstream for elimination, your mood or energy level may drop. You may feel cranky or irritable, but before you know it, the two days are over and you are eating solid food again. Food will taste so much better.

If you get hungry while fasting, rather than give it up, have a few little snacks to keep your blood sugar up. Ideal snacks would be about 25 calories and include protein, fat, and a little more carbohydrate. My favorite snack is three slices of an apple and three almonds. You could also cut up a popular balanced health bar into small pieces. I will also use chocolate or vanilla snacks by Isagenix, which contain a simple balance of nutrients to sustain healthy blood sugar. By having a little 25-calorie snack every two or three hours, you can get the maximum from fasting and avoid any hunger. Always follow your snack with 8 ounces of water. This will allow your body to absorb the nutrients and reduce hunger.

If you think it will be too difficult and you are not familiar with fasting, make sure you have a little snack every two hours. This will keep your blood sugar balanced and minimize food cravings. Try to stay active and entertained and avoid seeing food.

To activate and facilitate the cleansing response, avoid eating solid food (except the little snacks), and drink 8 ounces of water with lemon, minerals, honey, and aloe vera every hour instead. Drink this cleansing cocktail every hour, and then on the half hour, drink 8 ounces of pure water. After each cocktail, practice the bounce and shake breathing technique for two minutes. In addition, do the standard Mars and Venus morning exercise routine twice a day, once in the morning and once in the afternoon. This will help your body do what it is designed to do and will lessen the symptoms of detoxification.

Fasting is not for everyone and not necessary for children

under thirteen. It is not just a matter of willpower, but more important, one of preference. If you are satisfied losing 2 to 3 pounds a week, then just follow the regular Mars and Venus Diet and Exercise Program. Some people love food too much to think of going without it for two days. If two days seems too long, you could also do a modified seven-day version. Do a one-day fast at the beginning and end of the cycle instead of two days. You could also fast until sundown. Another option is to skip the fast and accelerate the normal Mars and Venus Solution by also replacing dinner with a shake. Using this formula, many of my friends and clients lost 5 to 6 pounds a week.

On this program, those with thyroid problems or a particularly low metabolism may only lose a half pound a day. Although this is much less than a pound a day, it is three times faster than other programs. So if you only lose a half pound a day, don't be discouraged.

THE DANGERS OF FAST WEIGHT LOSS

A pound a day is five times faster than most experts believe is possible. No wonder people get discouraged trying to lose weight. Most programs assist a person in losing only a pound and a half a week. When some experts hear this dramatic result, they can only assume that a diuretic or metabolic stimulants like ephedrine or ephedra, Fen-Phen, or ma-huang have been used. These stimulants also result in fast weight loss, but they are not healthy and the weight loss doesn't last.

Thirty years ago, there was a weight loss program that consisted of predigested proteins. This program provided accelerated weight loss, but the weight loss was primarily the loss of lean body mass. This definitely is not healthy.

Diuretic medications prescribed by a doctor can cause a person to lose 9 pounds in a couple of days. This loss is almost all water, and the weight will come back in a few days. Diuretics are not healthy, because they dehydrate your body rather than burn excess weight. You may weigh less, but you will gain it back very quickly.

This dramatic weight loss comes from burning fat and not water loss.

Many popular weight loss programs use ephedrine or ephedra and Fen-Phen to raise the metabolism to burn fat. What you eat does not matter. With a higher than normal metabolism, your body can and will burn whatever you put in it. People lose weight quickly, and they can eat lots of junk food. These programs are not safe because they put a strain on your heart. Some of these programs have been banned or are discouraged by experts.

Doctors have measured patients using the Mars and Venus accelerated Program and found that the weight loss is completely safe and results from burning fat. The loss is rapid only if you are overweight. If you are underweight, observing the same healing program will enable you to gain weight. Rather than a weight loss program, *The Mars and Venus Diet and Exercise Solution* is a healing program that results in accelerated healing. This program helps your body to heal itself no matter what the problem.

For gaining weight, the same cleansing program applies. After nine days, begin the normal Mars and Venus Diet and Exercise Program except add an hour a day of weight-bearing exercise. With a healthier liver and better nutrition coupled with regular weight-bearing exercise, you will give your body the support it needs to restore normal and healthy weight. To maintain your ideal weight, just follow the standard Mars and Venus Diet and Exercise Program.

10

HAVING A HEALTHY RELATIONSHIP WITH FOOD

Diets don't work because they require willpower. By willpower alone, you can carry a heavy weight for only so long, and then you have to put it down. In a similar manner, we can be motivated to avoid junk food for only so long, but then we go off our diets and once again begin eating refined sugar, processed foods, and hydrogenated oils. We can run on willpower for only so long. At a certain point, trying to follow a perfect diet becomes too much of a burden.

If your body is relatively healthy, you do not require perfect food all the time. Your body can cope with imperfection and actually grows stronger in that process. A healthy relationship with food is similar to a healthy relationship with life. Life will always challenge us to be more of who we truly are. Growth occurs through challenge. If everything were easy, we would not grow. You cannot expect to build muscle unless you challenge your muscles. Going to the gym and getting an easy weight to lift and then putting it down will not challenge your muscles, and they will not grow. Once you have challenged a muscle, it is important to give it plenty of rest to heal itself and grow.

If your soul wants to grow in love and everyone always loves you, then you will never be challenged to love in difficult circumstances. It is those moments of finding love when we don't feel loved that help us to grow in our ability to love more.

When our hearts have been wounded and we are able to return to love, forgiveness, and innocence, we grow in the real power of love. What gives us the ability to give more love than we are getting is the opportunity to receive love at other times. Ideally, in childhood, we get the love we need, and then for the rest of our lives, we derive our highest fulfillment from giving love. We still need to receive love, but our most important need is to give it.

In a similar manner, by having a healthy breakfast every day with all the nutrients that we need to create brain chemistry, we are then prepared to cope with life's stresses. Some of the stresses can be mistakes or imperfections in our diet. We should not plan to make mistakes, but we can learn from them. If our bodies are sick, we naturally are more motivated to eat a healthier diet. Once you restore your normal weight along with better health, you can be more free in what you eat.

In life, we should never plan to make mistakes, but as they occur, we can learn from them.

In our relationships, we should not seek out those who do not love us, but if this occurs and we are rejected, misunderstood, or not appreciated, we then have the opportunity to grow in love and character by returning to love through forgiveness, generosity, and compassion.

Ultimately, when you love yourself and forgive yourself for your mistakes, you are free to love others. Likewise, when you accept and forgive the shortcomings of others and seek to find the good in them, you are able to love yourself more. When we demand perfection of others, we demand that kind of perfection of ourselves.

LISTENING TO YOUR BODY

In a similar manner, when you have a healthy body, not only do you hunger for healthful food, but if you occasionally eat junk food, your body can deal with it and you don't gain weight or experience mood swings. When you eat the wrong foods, your body will tell you. Since you have learned to listen, you will not crave those foods as much. To listen to your body and learn from your experience, you must know what you are looking for.

Likewise, when we remind ourselves of what we are seeking, we can learn from our mistakes. By knowing what to expect from a healthy program, you will interpret the messages you get from your body more accurately.

Take a few minutes to set up some healthy expectations in the following guided meditations. Let each main idea sink into your subconscious mind, replacing the old outdated expectations. After reading each paragraph, close your eyes and recall what you read. By remembering the specific message, generate as best you can the experience in your mind, heart, and body. As you begin *The Mars and Venus Diet and Exercise Solution,* your goals will become more vivid and real each time you do this exercise.

GUIDED MEDITATIONS FOR A HEALTHY BODY

Exercise these eight levels of positive emotions, feelings, and attitudes with the following guided meditations:

1. Confident and relaxed. Imagine having an easy relationship with food, feeling confident and assured that you can eat what you want, because what you want is generally very good for your body and brain chemistry. You are relaxed about your diet because it is working for you. Every day you are getting healthier and happier. Your body and brain are getting what they need from the food you eat. Pause, close your eyes for a moment, and just feel this experience. When you open your eyes, move on to the next experience.

2. Joyful and motivated. Imagine being motivated each morning to do thirty minutes of enjoyable exercise. It becomes so enjoyable that you look for opportunities to do more. Instead of feeling sore or tired, you always get the immediate result of more energy and an endorphin rush to your brain. You feel comfortable in your body and with your body. As you begin to balance the levels of dopamine and serotonin in your brain, this dream will become a reality right away. Pause, close your eyes, and just feel this experience. When you open your eyes, move on to the next experience.

3. Free and abundant. Imagine being free of food cravings, simply eating what you want; what you want is in harmony with what you know is good for you. Feel like you can eat whatever you want and whenever you want. Only an imbalance in neural chemistry causes us to crave unhealthy foods; a healthy body hungers for healthful food and an unhealthy body craves food that is bad for us. Feel the relief that comes from enjoying healthy foods. Think about a healthy food combination that you like, and imagine eating it and enjoying every bite, then feeling completely satisfied. Pause, close your eyes, and just feel this experience. When you open your eyes, move on to the next experience.

4. Excited and enthusiastic. Imagine missing your healthy foods and wanting to taste them. Experience the feeling of excitement as you look forward to eating a delicious and healthy meal. What are the foods that you know are good for you? Experience yourself eating them on a regular basis and not only loving it, but loving how you feel afterwards. Pause, close your eyes, and just feel this experience. When you open your eyes, move on to the next experience.

5. Satisfied and content. Imagine having a big plate of delicious food in front of you and then feeling satisfied by eating only half of it. Although there is more food on your plate, you are completely satisfied and content with what you have already eaten. Give yourself time to enjoy your satisfaction, trusting that if you get hungry later, you can then eat again. Give your body the chance to digest what you have eaten and feel completely fulfilled. Imagine making the sound *ummm* and feeling completely satisfied. Pause, close your eyes, and feel this experience. When you open your eyes, move on to the next experience.

6. Flexible and in control. Imagine feeling vibrantly healthy and having the flexibility to eat unhealthy food occasionally because that is all that is available or because it would be fun. If you fall out of the zone of endless energy, experience forgiving yourself because you know you will reestablish the balance. If you have gained a few extra pounds, you are confident that within a couple of days, you will restore your body back to its ideal weight. You are in complete control of your weight. By adjusting your diet and returning to the zone of vibrant health, you will be able to burn whatever extra calories you have eaten. Pause, close your eyes, and feel that confidence and ease in your new relationship to food and weight. When you open your eyes, move on to the next experience.

7. Lovable and attractive. Imagine looking in the mirror and loving what you see. If you can remember a time when you liked what you saw, remember how that felt. If you have never loved your appearance, imagine how it would feel if your body was your ideal weight and you had perfect posture. Imagine seeing yourself standing up straight, with your ideal body in the mirror. Imagine how it would feel to love your body, overlooking its imperfections and appreciating its strengths. Pause, close your eyes, and feel the pleasure of loving yourself and feeling confident that your partner or future partner is attracted to you.

8. Healthier and happier. Imagine effortlessly getting up every day to do your morning exercises and enjoying the ease of making a highly nutritious breakfast shake in the morning. Every day your body is getting healthier, and you are feeling better and better. You have more energy, happiness, and love. Pause, close your eyes, and feel that confidence and ease in your new relationship to food and your body. When you open your eyes, take a long and deep breath. On the exhale, feel peaceful, confident, and complete.

Practice these guided meditations regularly, or record them on a tape and listen to it before bed or upon waking. By adjusting your expectations automatically, you will find it easier to achieve an easy transition to following your ideal diet and achieving brain balance. You can also get many of the same benefits just by reading the meditations again several times.

PRACTICE MAKES PERFECT

In the old school, practice makes perfect. Though this may be true in certain areas of life, it is not true when you consider the bigger picture. There are many people who achieve perfection in one area, but the rest of their life is a mess. To apply this program, don't seek to be perfect. Instead, try to find balance again when you inevitably go out of balance.

Most people know what a good diet is; they just have a hard time sticking to it. Though many diets may assist you in losing weight, they don't keep the weight off. Starting a new program, by virtue of its newness, will produce more dopamine.

For low-dopamine men, this in itself will make them work. Whenever a man does anything new, he will get the extra benefit of increased energy and motivation. If that diet doesn't give him the support to sustain that increased dopamine, he will lose interest after a while. He will get aroused, as he would in a new relationship, but that is no guarantee that it will last.

New diet programs and deprivation diets are
much easier for men to follow.

Women have more difficulty starting and staying on new diets, particularly if they are deprivation diets. If a woman says no all the time to what she wants, it decreases her levels of serotonin and increases her levels of dopamine. The increased dopamine will give her energy in the beginning, but if she doesn't have the support of her comfort foods, her serotonin drops and she will suffer food cravings. With their normally higher levels of serotonin, men do much better on deprivation diets. Eventually men feel they are missing something and stop.

The body will always seek balance. If you deprive yourself for a while, the pendulum will eventually swing the other direction, and you will seek to indulge your senses and binge on the very foods that you couldn't eat.

Ultimately, no diet can or will work unless it is supplemented with the nutrients the body needs not only to feed the cells but also to provide the right brain balance. Willpower may help you follow a diet for a few months or years, but inevitably your body will swing the other way and you will once again fall from grace and go off your diet.

Nothing in life is ever perfect. People who attempt to have a perfect diet or feel guilty for not staying on a perfect diet are destined to fail over and over again. Anyone who expects perfection will just be disappointed. Nothing in this world is perfect.

Is the weather perfectly sunny all the time?

Is the temperature perfect all the time?

Is anyone's mood perfect all the time?

Do you say the perfect thing all the time?

Do you always have the perfect answer to questions you are asked?

Do you always say, do, react, and respond in the perfect way to your children or spouse?

Do you always make perfect decisions at work or in your investments?

Does your partner always respond or react in the perfect manner?

I hope your answer to all of these questions is no. Nothing and no one in this world is perfect. Imperfection is part of our nature and reality. On one hand, our greatest joy and source of fulfillment is the movement toward more perfection. On the other hand, the expectation of or demand for perfection is our greatest block.

The biggest obstacle to staying happily married is the expectation that our partner be perfect. Our love life becomes so much easier when we stop wanting our partner to be the source of our fulfillment. For a relationship to work, we need to be educated in how to communicate our needs, thoughts, and feelings, but ultimately, it all comes down to our attitude. Are we expecting our partners to be perfect? Or are we able to accept their imperfections? With a more forgiving and accepting attitude, we are then able to open up and share our hearts.

Our love life becomes much easier when we stop demanding that we and others be perfect.

Likewise, staying on a healthy diet becomes much easier when we don't expect or require perfection. To stay healthy and happy and to experience lasting romance, we don't have to follow a perfect diet all the time. We can make mistakes and quickly recover. We can occasionally indulge ourselves and our senses, and then cleanse our systems and come back into balance.

Most people make the mistake of striving for perfection. When they cannot achieve it, they become discouraged and give up. They try again, and the cycle repeats itself. The Mars and Venus Solution helps you to break this cycle in all areas of your life.

THE SOLUTION: MOTIVATION

It is not enough to eat healthy food. The solution to sustaining a healthy diet is to eat foods that will create lasting motivation. It is our brain chemistry that keeps us motivated. Willpower that is not backed with energy and positive feelings can be sustained only temporarily. When we eat and exercise in a manner that promotes the right production of hormones and brain chemicals, we become more motivated. When the brain is motivated, healthy food actually tastes really good, and we want to eat it. When healthy foods are more satisfying, it is no longer an effort to choose them over junk food.

When the brain is motivated, healthy foods taste better.

Instead of trying to change what we eat, we should change what we *want* to eat. There are many things that can motivate us, but there is only one thing that can sustain that motivation. If we want to do something, then it is easy to do. By caring for our bodies through cleansing, supplementation, and exercise, we can stimulate the hormones in our bodies and brains to change our wants. With the correct brain chemistry, we can easily stay motivated to eat healthy and wholesome food.

Instead of trying to change what you eat, change what you *want* to eat.

Even with this sustained and automatic motivation, the option for occasionally skipping a meal, eating too much, or indulging in junk food is workable. The emphasis in *The Mars and Venus Diet and Exercise Solution* is always on supplementing what you eat with healthy nutrients. Adding, rather than trying to take away things, is not only much easier, it is healthier.

STAYING MOTIVATED

The first step of positive change is getting motivated. For most people, that is not a problem. So many motivational sources are available to us today. Never has so much information been available for improving our lives. Depending on experts, trainers, and coaches for motivation is not enough. Even having a personal trainer come to your house to motivate you, which is a great option for those who can afford it, is not enough. Inevitably your body, mind, and spirit will rebel!

If your diet and exercise program focuses on producing the brain chemistry of motivation, you will have discovered the missing key to sustain your healthy choices. When your body and brain are getting what they need, there is no feeling of deprivation. The need to rebel doesn't arise.

With sustained motivation, doing what is good and healthy for yourself is not a chore, burden, or effort. Changes that require sustained effort just don't last. If a change is easy and it produces results, then and only then will it be sustained for a lifetime.

If a change is easy and produces results, it can be sustained for a lifetime.

Motivation is everywhere. The key is staying motivated. Having correct brain chemistry doesn't mean that we don't also need good motivators. They are also an important part of the solution. Reading good books and exposing ourselves to people who have achieved what we want to achieve is essential to stay inspired. To stay healthy, we need to be connected to other people who are also health conscious.

We have all experienced the motivational influence of reading a good book, attending a spiritual gathering, participating in a church meeting, seeing a heartwarming movie, or listening to a passionate speaker. After these experiences, we feel great. We are suddenly motivated and enthusiastic to be all that we can be. The only drawback with motivational events is that the high dissipates.

WHY WE LOSE OUR MOTIVATION

Whenever we are inspired and motivated by others, a change occurs in our consciousness. We see ourselves and our lives in a different light. Suddenly we feel great. We look around and see that we are surrounded by opportunities to make our dreams come true. We see the bigger picture of ourselves and our lives.

We still recognize that there are problems, but we also have the power to overcome them and achieve our goals. Somehow, somewhere, there is a reason for it all. With every cell in our bodies, we sense the simple truth: We are in the right place at the right time, and we are doing what we are supposed to be doing. Everything is wonderful!

**When our consciousness changes,
we see a bigger picture of ourselves and our lives;
automatically, we are more motivated.**

This shift in our consciousness creates a change in brain and body. A motivated state of consciousness creates a motivated body. Not only are we feeling inspired, but our bodies feel energized as well. In this way the body and brain are intimately connected to our state of consciousness. When our consciousness changes, our bodies change.

**When our consciousness changes,
our bodies change as well.**

And it works the other way. When our bodies and brains change, our consciousness changes. That is why certain foods, herbs, or drugs have a dramatic effect on our mood, mental performance, and motivation. When drugs change brain chemistry, our thinking changes. When we eat certain foods or herbs to affect brain and body chemistry, our consciousness changes.

This is why diet can be so powerful to sustain a desired state of consciousness. If we eat a diet that supports the brain chemistry of motivation, then when we become motivated to make a change, our bodies will support that change, and we will be able to sustain our motivation.

**We can stay inspired
when we eat the right food.**

With a healthy diet, we can stay motivated! If we use our inspired state of consciousness to eat good foods that sustain healthy brain chemistry, the problem should be solved. Right? Well, not completely. If this was the absolute truth, everyone would be motivated to keep eating good and healthy food after eating a few healthy meals. Sounds good, but in reality it doesn't happen. There is another big factor in this equation.

THE PRINCIPLE OF PURIFICATION

When a change occurs in our consciousness, there is always a corresponding change in the body and brain. The cells in our bodies and brains immediately become more vibrant. They literally begin to vibrate faster. The whole body relaxes and says, "Okay, this is a better way of operating. I like this, I want to stay this way."

Here is the problem. To maintain this higher or more motivated state of consciousness, the body must purify itself to stay in this healthier and happier state of being. To uphold a higher state of consciousness, the body needs the right foods and nutrients, but it must also rid itself of the toxins associated with a less healthy style of functioning. It is not enough to eat foods that balance the production of brain chemicals. The body has to release old toxins as well. Let's explore this process of purification a little more deeply. It holds the secret to lasting change.

To uphold a higher state of consciousness, the body begins a process of purification.

When we get inspired, we think something like this: "I like this new way of thinking. I want to get rid of my old ways of thinking that don't serve me well. From this day onward, I release all the old thoughts and beliefs, like 'I can't do it' or 'I can't have that.' "

With greater understanding of a situation, we are able to release negative feelings and open our hearts again. We have thoughts like "I guess I can forgive that person. He just didn't know better. It's time to let go of my resistance and forgive. I suppose I can release this old hurt and anger." The process of emotional health is one of constantly learning from the past and then letting go of negative beliefs and feelings.

The body reacts to positive change in a similar manner. Instead of letting go of negative thoughts, feelings, and outdated beliefs, your body gets rid of stored toxins and accumulated viruses. Whenever you are inspired and moved to a higher state of consciousness, your body also shifts to a higher state of functioning. To sustain that higher consciousness, the cleansing process begins. The immune system becomes activated to lower the viral load. Millions of harmful bacteria, parasites, and viruses begin dying off. In addition, the lymphatic system and liver are activated to begin processing and releasing accumulated toxins.

When the mind is uplifted, the body begins to cleanse.

Imagine you won the lottery and suddenly had millions of dollars for the rest of your life. Next, you go out and buy a whole new wardrobe. When you come home, you now have a new chore. You have to clean out your closet to make room for all your new clothes. This is the principle of purification. You cannot avoid it. Whenever you make a positive mental change, your body needs to purify to uphold this change.

Sometimes the most positive and loving people have big guts to store their excess toxins, and even with lots of dieting and exercise, they can't lose this extra weight. These are often the people who have succeeded in elevating their consciousness, but have not learned the importance of helping out the liver with purification exercises. They are able to sustain their intention to be loving and kind, but their bodies are still holding on to stored toxins.

By understanding the principle of purification, we can clearly appreciate the value of cleansing to sustain higher consciousness.

Each time we make a positive mental change, toxins are released in the blood. If we do not assist the liver to process these toxins, then the body can become sick. To protect the liver and other organs from becoming toxic, the body returns to its original state before the shift in consciousness and stops the purification process.

To stop the release of more toxins, the body returns to its previous state before the shift in consciousness.

As our bodies go back to their previous state, our consciousness changes back as well. Our mood changes and our energy level drops. Suddenly we are back to where we started before we were motivated. Only now we have the burden of more guilt for not following through.

When too many toxins get released, the body does its best to protect you from all the toxins.

On Sunday, we are motivated, and on Monday, it is all gone. How many times have we resolved to make a change tomorrow and it did not happen? How many times are we motivated to be better, do better, eat better, and exercise better, only to fall back? To sustain our motivation, we need to find an effective way to purify our bodies, as well as eat the foods required to sustain higher brain functioning.

GIVING UP A BAD HABIT AND GETTING SICK

I remember helping one client give up smoking. He had been a smoker all his life. He was sixty-five years old and his children finally convinced him to stop smoking. His children didn't want him to die from lung cancer. It was very difficult, but motivated by the love of his children, he did it. Three weeks after he quit, he began to develop a tumor in his throat. He couldn't believe it. He had given up a deadly habit, and as a result he had started getting deadly sick.

He decided that if he was going to die of throat cancer, he would start smoking again and die happier. Within a few weeks, the tumor went away. He couldn't believe it. It just didn't make sense.

Once he understood the principle of purification, it all became clear. Giving up smoking had caused his body to release so many toxins that he got sick. He didn't drink more water or exercise in a manner to help the body release all the old, accumulated toxins from years of smoking. When he started smoking again, his body stopped releasing toxins and the tumor went away.

Getting sick after giving up a bad habit doesn't always happen, because people often replace one bad habit with another. When alcoholics give up drinking, they often replace drinking with another addiction, like overeating sugar, drinking too much coffee, or smoking. Without the option of an efficient cleansing program, going from one toxic habit to another, less toxic habit is actually much healthier than giving up every bad habit all at once.

FOOD SUPPLEMENTS FOR CLEANSING

When I was in Dr. Hitt's clinic, I was repeatedly amazed by the dramatic benefits of purifying the blood through intravenous ozone therapy. When you put more oxygen in the blood, the viral load is decreased, your immune system is significantly strengthened, and your body is purified of toxic viruses. Though this treatment is highly effective, you will get many of the same benefits at home every morning by drinking your activated water before and after your ten- to thirty-minute Mars and Venus exercise routine.

By drinking a glass of water with lemon juice, minerals, aloe vera, and honey when you first get up in the morning, you can greatly assist your liver and lymphatic system in the daily process of cleansing. A cleaner system supports your mental consciousness and your body's immune system.

With the Mars and Venus Solution, you will activate your lymphatic system to cleanse your way to better health by giving up one bad habit at a time. By making sure you help your body cleanse itself every morning, you will be able to sustain your motivation to eat healthier foods. With sustained motivation, you will make whatever diet you choose work for you.

11

THE MARS AND VENUS PROTEIN AND FAT EQUATION

A healthy diet requires the right quantity, quality, and balance of nutrients. Different diet programs tend to focus on one of these three ingredients. The Mars and Venus Program includes all three, as well as the best food choices for your sex and body type. Descriptions of diets rarely ever mention our gender differences, and very few people understand how our body type affects our dietary needs for producing correct brain chemistry and weight management. In this chapter we explore the right quantity, quality, and balance of nutrients for our sex.

By consuming a low-calorie, nutrient-dense, balanced breakfast shake every morning, you won't have to worry and fuss about eating a perfect diet during the day. With a basic understanding of the right quantity, quality, and balance of nutrients, eating a healthy diet the rest of the day will be increasingly effortless. First, let's cover the basic elements of a healthy Mars and Venus diet.

QUANTITY OF NUTRIENTS

With the right quantity of calories for breakfast, your body will start out functioning at peak performance. You will not be burdened and exhausted by having to digest too much food. With more efficient digestion and assimilation of nutrients for the rest of the day, you don't have to worry about counting calories to determine the right quantity. Your body will just tell you how much you need to eat. You will be surprised that most of the time you will not even want to finish the food on your plate.

If you don't want to rely solely on your hunger to tell you, a simple way to measure the right amount of food for you is a portion the size of your hand. Make your protein portion at lunch and dinner about the size you could easily hold in your palm.

Depending on your current weight, you will need between 200 and 300 calories of food for breakfast. If you are already at your ideal weight, you can eat more if you like. If you are overweight, a low-calorie but nutrient-dense breakfast tells your body to burn extra body fat for more energy. If you are concerned about this, consider that the healthy Hunza population have an extremely low-calorie breakfast and live well beyond a hundred without suffering from our common Western diseases.

If your ideal weight is less than 135 pounds, eat 200 calories. If your ideal weight is more than 200 pounds, eat a maximum of 300 calories. If your ideal weight is between 135 and 200 pounds, then multiply your ideal weight by 1.5.

For example, if your ideal weight is 150 pounds, then eat approximately 225 calories for breakfast ($150 \times 1.5 = 225$).

This is a good working start. If you wish to increase or lower your calorie amount, do so. Always listen to your body in making the right adjustments for you.

QUALITY OF NUTRIENTS

If you have high quality nutrients in the morning, the quality of food you eat during the day will not be as important. Your tastes will change, and you will naturally be attracted to healthier food. Your craving for junk food will disappear.

Just do your best to eat whole, unprocessed foods, fresh vegetables, and fruit whenever possible, and free-range or low-fat, lean animal products. The fat in animal products and in eggs is changed when animals are not allowed to eat grass. Grain-fed animals raised without the opportunity to walk around all day produce fat deficient in the essential fatty acid called omega-3. Omega-3 fat is essential for producing dopamine and serotonin in the brain.

The fat in animal products and in eggs is changed when animals are not allowed to eat grass.

Good Fats Versus Bad Fats

Research over the past five years reveals that an increase in omega-3 dietary fat produces a long list of benefits, including a decrease in PMS symptoms in women and less depression in both men and women. Eating omega-3 fatty acid supplements has been shown to accelerate weight loss. Free-range animal products will always be your healthiest choice. Though free-range animal products cost more, they are worth it. Your fast food choices do not come from free-range animals.

Eating omega-3 fatty acid supplements has been shown to accelerate weight loss.

If you are a vegetarian, just make sure that you are getting enough complete proteins in your grains and legumes. You will generally need to eat a variety of grains and beans to get a complete protein. Without a complete protein combination at every meal, your brain cannot make sufficient amounts of brain chemicals.

For vegetarians and nonvegetarians, an abundance of healthy vegetables is essential. Meat and potatoes or rice and beans (a complete protein combination) are not enough. More vegetables are good for everyone. Organic vegetables and foods are less likely to contain harmful chemicals and have more of the minerals and vitamins your body desperately needs.

Processed foods are depleted of minerals, enzymes, and vitamins. Cooking regular or organic food kills their life-giving enzymes. To get enough enzymes, try to eat more raw foods like nuts, dried fruits, carrots, tomatoes, lettuce, and celery. Whenever you can add them to a meal, do it. The darker the lettuce, the more healthy minerals it will contain. If you don't eat enough raw foods or high quality organic food, boost your food with enzyme and mineral supplements.

Even a few raw foods are better than nothing. Eat raw foods at the beginning of the meal to give your body enough enzymes. Chew raw foods more thoroughly to activate your body's ability to use these enzymes. Digestion starts in the mouth.

Eat raw foods at the beginning of the meal to give your body enough enzymes to digest the rest.

Whole books have been written on good fats and bad fats. My favorites and the easiest for me to understand are *Eat Fat, Lose Weight* by Ann Louise Gittleman and *The Schwarzbein Principle* by Diana Schwarzbein. They not only dispel the myth that fat is bad but confirm that some fats are really good for you. The bad fats are in processed foods. They are identified on food labels as hydrogenated fats. Adding hydrogen to fats extends the shelf life of an oil. When an oil or fat can't go rancid on the shelf, that means your stomach cannot digest it. It is not only useless to the body; it is toxic. Hydrogenated fats are also called trans fats.

Research has shown that trans fats contribute to impaired cellular function, clogged arteries, and degenerative disease. When you eat bad fats, your body doesn't recognize them and is unable to process them or benefit from them. They are believed to interfere with the body's ability to process good fats efficiently. These trans fats are very common in our modern Western diet.

For example, all deep-fried foods and margarine contain

these harmful fats. The fats in deep-fried foods have been transformed into trans fats by cooking at high temperatures. The unwanted trans-fatty acids in margarine and shortening are two of the most damaging fatty substances you can eat.

These are some of the foods with trans-fatty acids that you want to minimize or avoid: bottled salad dressings, deep-fat-fried foods, high-fat meats cooked at high temperatures (order rare to medium rare), hydrogenated oils, imitation mayonnaise, imitation sour cream, lard or shortening, nondairy creamers, pressurized whipped cream (the real thing is much better for you), and all processed foods and fast foods that use hydrogenated oils. French fries and doughnuts are fun foods, but keep them to a minimum because they are toxic to your body. If you crave junk food, eat a healthier choice such as ice cream, chocolate, or one of the popular health bars: PowerBar, Zone Bar, Luna Bar, or Balance Bar.

French fries and doughnuts are fun foods but keep them to a minimum because they are toxic to your body.

Most experts agree that we are deficient in omega-3 fatty acids. Many research programs have demonstrated that one or two tablespoons a day of flaxseed oil have a profound effect on health, energy levels, and stabilizing moods. You can also mix flax oil with olive oil for a great-tasting salad dressing. The Mars and Venus breakfast solution includes dietary fat from flaxseeds or hemp seeds, which are naturally rich in omega-3 fatty acids.

Simple Carbs and Complex Carbs

There are basically two types of carbohydrates: simple and complex. Simple carbohydrates are the sugars, mainly table sugar and other natural sweeteners, the fructose in fruit, and the lactose in milk. Complex carbohydrates are found in starches, grains, legumes, and vegetables. Both simple and complex carbs break down into glucose for the body to use. The big difference is that simple sugars are released much faster into the bloodstream.

The brain needs a constant supply of sugar in the blood. If there is not enough sugar, you will have low energy and foggy thinking. Too much is not good, either. The pancreas releases insulin to lower blood sugar. Too much sugar results in a quick high and then a low. To avoid this emotional roller coaster, eat more complex carbs. They are released much more slowly into the blood, and they are healthier.

Carbs that are released quickly into the blood are high on what is called the glycemic index, and healthier foods that release more slowly are low on the glycemic index. On pages 253-254 is a list of high and low glycemic foods.

When choosing your carbohydrates, keep in mind these points:

• Natural fructose (the sugar from fruit) is better because it releases into the blood much more slowly than other refined sugars and natural sweeteners. It must be processed by the liver before the sugar is released into the blood. Other simple sugars go straight into the blood and can easily cause mood swings, hyperactivity, and weight gain.

• When proteins and fats are eaten with high glycemic foods, they help slow down the absorption of sugar and prevent sharp rises in blood sugar.

• Energy levels are linked to the foods you eat. High glycemic foods (simple sugars) give you a burst of energy, but let you down. Foods lower on the glycemic index provide a long-term supply of energy.

• Refined carbohydrates (simple or complex) lack the vitamins, minerals, and fiber that whole foods possess. These refined products deplete your body of stored minerals and vitamins.

Eating refined or processed carbohydrates increases the glycemic release and results in food cravings. These cravings can put you out of balance, making you want to eat more than you need. With a balanced breakfast, this impulse will weaken. Whenever possible, eat fewer refined and processed foods to maintain steady and healthy blood sugar levels. Steady blood sugar means unending energy. If you are experiencing drops in your energy in the afternoon after eating, it is the result of low blood sugar.

BALANCE OF NUTRIENTS

With a balanced breakfast shake every morning, you will get the precise amounts of protein, carbohydrates, and dietary fat your body needs. This exact proportion is easily measured out every morning by adding exact amounts of specific ingredients in your morning shake according to the Mars and Venus formula.

We have already discussed that for the ideal production of brain chemistry, both men and women need about 50 percent carbohydrates. Men need 30 percent protein and 20 percent fat, and women need 20 percent protein and 30 percent fat. With this Mars and Venus balance, you will have the perfect combination to create healthy brain chemistry.

Men need 30 percent protein and 20 percent fat, and women need 20 percent protein and 30 percent fat.

More protein for men and less for women ensures that men get enough protein to produce dopamine and that women don't get too much protein, which could inhibit serotonin production. More fat in the diet creates more oxytocin, which is particularly good for women; more protein creates more testosterone, which is good for men. When a woman's diet is deficient in good fats, she craves too much food. When men don't get enough protein or can't digest the proteins they consume, they eat too much as well.

More fat in the diet creates oxytocin for women;
more protein creates testosterone for men.

More fat for women stimulates the production of prostaglandins, which help to balance her hormones and stimulate the production of more serotonin. Women are born with more fat receptor cells, because their hormone requirements are greater than a man's. More fat for men creates too much serotonin, and can result in sleepiness and low energy.

In this context, more fat means women require more fat than men. Both men and women need to be careful to keep their overall fat intake lower. It is true that Americans eat too much fat, but fat generally gets a bad rap. Without a solid low-calorie breakfast in the morning, most people overeat all nutrients, not just fat. It is not too much fat that causes heart disease, diabetes, and high blood pressure. Eating too much of *all* the nutrients does.

A study of 12,000 men surveyed in seven countries revealed that the men on the Greek island of Crete were significantly healthier than the men studied in Italy, the Netherlands, Finland, Yugoslavia, Japan, and the United States. In his book *The Omega Diet,* Dr. Artemis P. Simopoulos presents this miraculous Crete diet. The program has proven to have tremendous healing results for people with cancer and heart disease, as well as for weight and stress management. On the island of Crete, the dietary fat intake is often 40 percent of total calories!

In his book *Enter the Zone,* Barry Sears helped to release our society from the grip of fat fear. He points out, in a very clear and convincing manner, the importance of balancing carbohydrates, proteins, and fats. He recommends a 40/30/30 percentage balance of carbs, proteins, and fats. Many world-class athletes are recognizing the importance of increasing their fat intake to 30 percent and their endurance has improved.

Any percentage of fat, even if you are eating good fats, is very unhealthy if you are *overeating* at every meal. Overweight, skinny, and even perfectly sculpted Americans typically eat twice as many calories as they need to eat. The fats they eat may even be a healthy 20 to 40 percent, but they are eating twice as much as they need. In this case, it is the quantity and not the balance that is killing Americans.

In researching the diverse diets and programs, one can easily conclude that a diet of 20 to 40 percent good fats, rich in omega-3 fatty acids, has been proven beyond a doubt to be healthy. So relax and enjoy more good fat in your food.

BALANCING YOUR DIET

Like a doctor administering the precise amounts of your medicine each morning, you will be feeding your body a perfect balance of nutrients to start the day. You will activate your metabolism for the rest of the day and stimulate the production of brain chemicals, so that during the day you will naturally hunger for a balanced diet.

During the day, all you have to do at your regular meals is make sure you have *about* equal amounts of calories from protein, carbohydrates, and dietary fat. If your nutrients are basically good quality, then you can eat as much as you want.

If you are eating processed foods, you may need to use a little willpower. Processed foods are nutritionally deficient and make you hungrier than you really are.

Processed foods are nutritionally deficient and
make you hungrier than you really are.

If you know you are eating too much and you have difficulty eating less, here are six strategies to help you stop:

1. Eat very slowly, and tell yourself if you leave food on your plate, you will get dessert. In restaurants, people sometimes feel

obligated to finish the food on their plates to avoid insulting the cook. Just say you are saving room for dessert. By waiting for dessert, you can easily stop eating. When you order dessert, offer to share it with others, and don't feel that you have to finish it.

2. Remove the food from your sight and go for a walk. Make a deal with yourself. If you are still hungry after the walk, you can eat more. Even a short walk to the bathroom could do the trick.

3. Stop eating, drink a glass of water with lemon, and then see if you still need to eat.

4. Stop eating, drink a glass of water with lemon, and then have a dessert treat, or promise yourself that later you will have a treat if you are still hungry. Lemon will help keep your blood sugar low so that you don't crave more sweets.

5. Stop eating, drink a glass of water with lemon, and then promise yourself that in one hour you can finish the meal if you are still hungry.

6. Have snacks or a low-calorie nutrient-dense shake between meals and make sure not to miss a meal. If you skip lunch, it is very difficult not to overeat at dinner. In this case, drinking a shake before dinner will help a lot to avoid overeating.

**If you know you are eating too much,
stop by promising yourself a treat in an hour
if you are still hungry.**

Keep in mind during the day that the balance of your foods doesn't have to be precise or perfect. Just make sure to include a portion of protein, carbohydrate, and dietary fat. As another general guideline, men need bigger portions of protein and women need a little more dietary fat. If the balance is not perfect, don't worry about it. It is so easy to become fanatical about balance. Nowhere in life do we experience perfect balance; why should we expect it in our diet?

Just make sure at every meal you include all of the three basic nutrients: protein, carbohydrate, and dietary fat. Here are some of my favorites. They are good examples of balancing your nutrients.

• If you are having a bagel or toast, make sure you add a little salmon, chicken, or tuna for protein. Also add some butter or cream cheese for the dietary fat. Add a little lettuce to get some raw food. Remember, cooking foods kills the enzymes. If you are eating only cooked food, take enzyme supplements with your meal.

• If you want a light meal, just have two pieces of sprouted hemp bread with butter and jam. It has all the protein you need for a light meal, plus a good supply of omega-3 dietary fat. Add some butter and jam for taste, and you have a complete meal. Or you could melt some mozzarella on top and add a slice of tomato. This is the healthiest pizza you could ever eat. Hemp bread also has a lot of fiber to keep you regular. I eat hemp bread as a treat almost every day.

• If you are having a baked potato, which is a high-carbohydrate, high glycemic food, then add some cheese, butter, or sour cream for dietary fat. Add bacon or soy bacon bits for protein. Add some green chives to get your enzymes. In this way, you will be creating a balance of essential nutrients. Women particularly benefit from sweet potatoes or yams with butter and some protein on the side. In Japan, women commonly eat sweet potatoes for breakfast. Sweet potatoes are very good for producing serotonin in the morning. There is no word for PMS or hot flash in Japanese.

• If you have a salad for lunch, make sure to add generous portions of healthy virgin olive oil for your dietary fat and some protein such as chicken, salmon, eggs, or turkey.

• If you have a bowl of rice, oatmeal, or buckwheat, which are all carbohydrates, add one or two cooked eggs on top. The egg whites have plenty of protein, and the yolk has the fat your body needs. Whenever possible, have omega-3 eggs. Try eating cooked quinoa as an alternative. Add green or red grapes, chopped onions, parsley, and goat cheese to cold quinoa for a great salad treat.

• If you are having toast and jam and the bread is not high-protein hemp bread, add a generous portion of peanut butter or almond butter for your protein and fat. Nuts are all high in protein and fat. Since they are raw, you will be getting some enzymes.

• For a snack, I often enjoy a couple of tablespoons of crunchy almond butter, apple slices, and a little honey. What a great mixture!

• If you are having fruit, balance this healthy fructose carbohydrate with a handful of your favorite nuts.

• If you are having a meat and potato meal, make sure to start with a salad. A salad will provide some raw food, which gives you enough enzymes to digest your cooked meal. Healthy olive oil on your salad will activate your body's fat-burning ability and its ability to process amino acids much better than animal fat. In this way, you will be giving your body what it needs to produce the brain chemistry of health and happiness.

• If you are having a dessert treat with refined sugar, make sure that it is after a meal. The fat and protein in your stomach will slow down the release of sugar into your bloodstream, reducing the chances of high blood sugar.

• If you eat dessert, make sure it has a balance of protein, fat, and carbohydrate. For example, peaches are the carb and cream has protein and fat. Add a few nuts for more protein, and you have a healthier dessert. If you eat ice cream, add some nuts and you will have a better balance.

• If you eat sushi, make sure to balance the fat and protein of raw or cooked fish with the rice. Add the seaweed and you get a lot of good minerals. Fermented miso soup helps your body kill parasites that may be in the raw fish. My favorite is tuna sushi. It contains lots of omega-3 fat. Eating fish raw gives your body all the enzymes it needs for digestion. Salmon, tuna, mackerel, and sardines contain the most omega-3 of all fishes.

• If you are having eggs in the morning, balance that protein with carbohydrates and fats by making a cheese omelet with plenty of your favorite vegetables. Zucchini, yellow summer squash, bell peppers, mushrooms, onions, tomatoes, asparagus, and broccoli are great additions.

- One of my favorite quick meals is a quesadilla. Melt mozzarella on a whole wheat or corn tortilla, and add salsa and slices of avocado. Add a slice of turkey or chicken for more protein. If you have more time to prepare, add some canned black beans and a couple of fried eggs to go on top.

Ultimately, just as important as balance is the quality and quantity of each nutrient. You could have the perfect balance but too many calories, and your brain chemistry will go out of balance, creating a craving for unhealthy foods. You could have the perfect balance and the correct number of calories, but the quality of foods you put in your body could be nutritionally deficient in minerals, vitamins, good fats, complete proteins, and good carbohydrates.

EATING TO BALANCE BLOOD SUGAR

To increase the amount of serotonin and dopamine in the brain, we need an abundance of carbohydrates. At the same time, we must be careful to keep our blood sugar balanced. When blood sugar is too high, insulin is released to lower blood sugar. With lower levels of blood sugar, the brain lessens its production of brain chemicals. To keep your blood sugar balanced, eat less high glycemic food and more low glycemic complex carbohydrates.

Low glycemic carbohydrates promote the steady uptake of tryptophan and increase serotonin action. With the right balance of protein, men produce plenty of dopamine.

High glycemic foods are not bad, but they should be eaten in moderation. Eat them in combination with the right balance and quantity of proteins and fats. If you are more sugar-sensitive, make sure you eat fewer high glycemic foods and more fat.

Cookies, for example, are high on the glycemic list, but ice cream is lower on the list. This is because the fat in ice cream slows down the release of sugar into the bloodstream. If a food is high on the glycemic list and you eat a small amount of it, this is better for your blood sugar than eating a lot of another food that is low on the list. For most people, one cookie is not the problem. Eating the whole bag is what causes your blood sugar to skyrocket.

Here is a list of carbohydrates rated from high to low on the glycemic list. Keep in mind that by balancing your carbohydrates with proteins and fats, you lower their glycemic level.

Almost Off the Charts
White bread and other white-flour products
Pastries, doughnuts, and sweet rolls
Mashed or instant potatoes
Candy bars, chocolate, and cookies
Processed fruit sugar (added sugar)
White and instant rice
Corn chips
Puffed rice and rice cakes

High
Cornflakes and other processed breakfast cereals
Raisins and other dried fruits
Baked, boiled, and french fried potatoes
Bananas, mangoes, apricots, pineapples, watermelon
Cooked carrots
Refined pastas
Honey

Moderate
Whole wheat bread and other whole grain products
Brown rice
Whole grain cereals without sugar
Couscous
Beets
Applesauce

Orange and grapefruit juice
Whole/mixed grain pasta
Corn
Sweet potatoes and yams
Green peas
Grapes, oranges, peaches, blueberries
Lentil and split pea soup
Instant noodles and macaroni
Popcorn, tortilla chips, and potato chips
Custard

Low
Leafy green vegetables
Yogurt (low-fat, unsweetened)
Kidney, black, and brown beans
Split peas and black-eyed peas
Lentils
Chickpeas
Apples, pears, plums, cherries, grapefruit
Soybeans
Tomatoes
Mushrooms
Peanuts
Ice cream (Yes, that's right; the fat content in ice cream
   lowers its glycemic rating.)
Fructose
Whole milk and skim milk

Really Low
Soybeans
Peanuts

EATING TO PRODUCE SEROTONIN FOR WOMEN

To produce more serotonin, you can combine this method of eating to balance your blood sugar with selecting specific proteins that are already high in their levels of tryptophan. What follows is a list of proteins that have relatively higher levels of tryptophan when compared with phenylalanine and leucine levels. When tryptophan doesn't have to compete with higher levels of phenylalanine and leucine, the uptake of tryptophan is greater and serotonin levels are higher. Phenylalanine is primarily responsible for producing dopamine and inhibits serotonin production. The amino acid leucine decomposes tryptophan. The ideal serotonin-producing foods have a higher SPF rating: SPF = serotonin production factor = tryptophan/(phenylalanine + leucine).

As we explore this list of high SPF foods, keep in mind that these are also great foods for men. They are just particularly useful for women to eat. Here is a list of the top fifty-four serotonin-producing foods.

Food	SPF Rating
1. Parsley	1.00
2. Edible boletus (porcini mushrooms)	.98
3. Seaweed—kelp (kombu)	.40
4. Dried dates	.35
5. Papaya	.31
6. Chanterelle mushrooms	.29
7. Cassava (yucca)	.29
8. Tapioca	.29
9. Beer	.25
10. Onions	.24
11. Portobella mushrooms	.23
12. Mushrooms	.22
13. Pecans	.21
14. Mustard greens	.20
15. Watermelon	.20
16. Celery	.20
17. Yellow mustard seed	.20
18. Rutabaga	.19
19. Spirulina	.19
20. Seaweed—wakame	.18
21. Winter squash	.18

Food	SPF Rating
22. Carrots	.18
23. Turnips	.18
24. Beets	.18
25. Dried apricots	.17
26. Sweet peppers	.17
27. Oranges	.17
28. Mangoes	.17
29. Milk whey	.16
30. Apricots, strawberries, tangerines	.16
31. Cherries, pineapple, and plums	.16
32. Grapefruit	.16
33. Butter	.16
34. Hot chili peppers	.16
35. Beets	.16
36. Sunflower seeds	.16
37. Hot peppers	.15
38. Sweet potatoes	.15
39. Squash	.15
40. Pumpkin	.15
41. Guava	.14
42. Chocolate	.14
43. Tomato paste	.14
44. Buckwheat	.14
45. Asian pears	.13
46. Almonds	.13
47. Tomatoes	.13
48. Pumpkin seeds	.13
49. Sesame seeds	.13
50. Potatoes	.13
51. Brussels sprouts	.13
52. Whole wheat flour	.13
53. Figs	.12
54. Bananas, grapes	.11

EATING TO PRODUCE DOPAMINE FOR MEN

To produce more dopamine, you need to be a little more careful with high glycemic foods. Not only do they lessen production of brain chemicals, but they will produce a spike in serotonin, which tends to lower a man's levels of dopamine. Eating more protein and fewer high glycemic carbohydrates will help keep a man's or boy's blood sugar stable so that his brain can produce dopamine and not too much serotonin. To ensure dopamine production, eat foods that are high in protein and low in fat. Too much fat inhibits the production of dopamine.

These are some proteins that are low in fat. Keep in mind that these proteins are also great foods for women. They are just particularly useful for men to eat. Here is a list of the top fifty-five high-protein, low-fat, dopamine-producing foods. To the side of each is the percentage of fat relative to protein. The ideal fat-to-protein relationship in a meal is 68 percent for men and 150 percent for women. If a rating is 100 percent, that means there is an equal amount of fat- and protein-burning calories. As we have already discussed, women are born with more fat cells and require more dietary fat.

Food	Fat-to-Protein Ratio (%)
1. Egg whites	0 (all protein and no fat)
2. Whey	0–2.5
3. Adzuki, kidney, lima, and mung beans	2–10
4. Crab	6
5. Cod	8
6. Flounder	9
7. Skim milk	9
8. Abalone	9
9. Lobster	10
10. Clams	15

Food	Fat-to-Protein Ratio (%)
11. Black beans	15
12. Low-fat cottage cheese	16
13. Shrimp	19
14. Sea bass	25
15. Turkey (light meat without skin)	25
16. Halibut	25
17. Spirulina	31
18. Chicken (light meat without skin)	33
19. Refried beans	36
20. Wheatberry English muffin	37
21. Swordfish	44
22. English muffin	45
23. Liver (beef and chicken)	45
24. Slice of lean ham	50
25. Yellowtail tuna	50
26. Sprouted flax bread	57
27. Turkey (dark meat without skin)	57
28. Tuna	63
29. Low-fat yogurt	64
30. Salmon	70
31. Custard-style yogurt	75
32. Oysters	75
33. Lean T-bone steak	80
34. Low-fat milk	81
35. Lean lamb	81
36. Chicken (dark meat without skin)	83
37. Oatmeal	83
38. Scallops	90
39. Tempeh	90
40. Duck (without skin)	100
41. Sardines	112
42. Tofu	112
43. Lentils	112

Food	Fat-to-Protein Ratio (%)
44. Boiled green soybeans	122
45. Soybean nuts	122
46. Low-fat mozzarella	129
47. Chicken (dark meat with skin)	141
48. Extra-lean ground beef	144
49. Mackerel	150
50. Turkey sausage	150
51. Chicken or turkey hot dog	160
52. Chicken noodle soup	162
53. Whole egg	200
54. Regular ground beef	205
55. Whole yogurt	209

All grains—barley, buckwheat, corn, millet, rye, wheat, for example—have moderate levels of protein and very little fat. They are a healthful low-fat staple for both men and women. On the other end of the spectrum are high-fat protein foods that should be eaten with caution. Here is a list of high-protein and high-fat foods to use in moderate portions.

Food	Fat-to-Protein Ratio (%)
56. Swiss cheese (and most other cheese)	218
57. Whole milk	225
58. Regular T-bone steak	270
59. Cheddar cheese	297
60. Feta cheese	330
61. Bacon	350
62. Sausage	360
63. Peanut butter	401

Food	Fat-to-Protein Ratio (%)
64. Ribs	472
65. Peanuts	487
66. Almonds	525
67. Beef bologna	545
68. Cashews (most nuts are high in fat)	675
69. Pecans	1,866
70. Macadamia nuts	1,875

There is nothing wrong with high-fat protein as long as it is in small portions and balanced with some nonfat protein. We have already discussed that fat is good, but not in amounts more than 20 to 40 percent of the total calories in a meal. For example, a few macadamia nuts are fine, but count them as your fat requirement rather than your protein requirement.

EATING MORE OMEGA-3 EFAs

Eating more protein will inhibit serotonin for women, so to keep blood sugar levels balanced, a woman needs to rely more on good fats to slow down the release of high glycemic carbohydrates. With plenty of protein to reduce the glycemic index of carbohydrates, men still need these good fats to produce brain chemicals. Men need more of the omega-3 essential fatty acids and fewer omega-6, as do women, but men require smaller quantities. Below is a list of foods high in omega-3 essential fatty acids and low in omega-6. By eating more omega-3, we can restore the right balance in our bodies.

1. Various cold-water fish: salmon, mackerel, cod, and tuna
2. Sea vegetables such as nori, hijiki, and kombu
3. Walnuts
4. Pumpkin seeds

5. Soybeans
6. Kidney beans
7. Flaxseeds and flaxseed oil
8. Hemp seeds and hemp seed oil
9. Cod liver oil

HYDROGENATED FATS TO AVOID OR MINIMIZE

As we have discussed, trans fats and hydrogenated oils are to be avoided. Treat them as you would junk food. They can be found in most junk foods. Take time to check labels for hydrogenated fats. Higher quality cookies, chips, and so forth are made without these harmful fats. Companies tend to hydrogenate fats to extend the shelf life of their products. Many food developers know that hydrogenated fats make food more addictive. Here is a list of foods high in hydrogenated fats:

1. Margarine
2. Cookies
3. White bread
4. Candies
5. Cakes
6. Doughnuts
7. Chips

FOODS HIGH IN SATURATED FATS

Fats that are solid at room temperature, such as butter and vegetable shortening, are called saturated fats. Much research has shown that too much saturated fat increases the risk of heart disease and obesity. This risk is minimized when we balance our omega-3 and omega-6 essential fatty acids. By supplementing our diet with fats high in omega-3, we do not have to worry as much about eating too much saturated fat.

Eating an excess of foods high in saturated fats will inhibit your energy levels, motivation, and clarity. Studies show that high-fat foods cause a decline in alertness and concentration. Too much saturated fat inhibits dopamine production. To get the benefit of creating healthy brain chemistry, eat lean meats in moderate amounts. Here is a list of foods high in saturated fats:

1. Beef
2. Pork
3. Lamb
4. Luncheon meats
5. Sausage
6. Hot dogs
7. Butter
8. Mayonnaise
9. Ice cream
10. Cream cheese
11. Egg yolks
12. Cheese
13. Whole milk and dairy products
14. Coconut

PICKING YOUR COOKING OILS

Unfortunately, we tend to get many of our essential fatty acids (EFAs) from sources such as cooking oils. Most cooking oils derived from nuts, seeds, and grains have relatively high concentrations of omega-6 and no omega-3. *Vegetable oil* sounds really healthy, but it is not. This includes oils derived from safflower, sunflower, corn, and peanuts. Better oils are derived from rapeseed (canola oil), soybeans, and sesame seeds. They have lower levels of omega-6 and relatively higher levels of omega-3.

Vegetable oil sounds really healthy, but it is not.

Olive oil is well known for its healthy properties. Greeks eat a diet rich in olive oil and have the lowest death rates from heart disease in the world. Research shows that women who take olive oil daily have a 25 percent less chance of developing breast cancer. The list of benefits goes on and on. Many experts conclude that extra virgin cold-pressed olive oil is the best of the common brands. Olive oil doesn't have much omega-3, but it has low levels of omega-6. By lessening your intake of omega-6, you are also helping to restore a healthy balance of omega-3 to omega-6. We already get too many omega-6 EFAs from our high intake of meats, eggs, fish, and dairy products.

The best oils for cooking when considering the production of brain chemistry are olive oil and sesame seed oil. Canadian-made canola oil, which is also good for cooking, has higher levels of omega-3 and low levels of omega-6, but many think that it is overprocessed.

Canola oil, which is also good for cooking, has higher levels of omega-3 and low levels of omega-6.

Many experts consider Canadian-made canola oil to be healthier than American brands. Canola oil was invented in Canada, from which it derived its name. Canadians produce a high quality oil that is not overly processed. I personally use and recommend most oils prepared by Spectrum in California.

When considering all the fats you are eating, avoid using oil to cook your food whenever possible. Broil, grill, bake, or barbecue your meats and fish, and steam your vegetables whenever possible.

Ghee, or clarified butter, is commonly used in India. Its advantage over butter is that it does not burn at high temperatures. Indian folklore attributes many healing properties to ghee. It has practically no omega-6 or omega-3, but it is high in calories, so don't overdo it. Butter is also good.

Many nutritionists are now recommending coconut oil as an alternative for cooking or spreading on your toast, replacing your need for butter and other oils. In the past, coconut oil, which is high in saturated fat, was associated with increasing levels of cholesterol. This early research was done on hydrogenated coconut oil, which is a trans fat and bad for you. Nonhydrogenated coconut oil is now available and has many impressive health-giving qualities.

Numerous studies show that coconut oil is high in lauric acid. Lauric acid is a chemical found in human mother's milk that is beneficial in attacking viruses, bacteria, and other pathogens, and is known for its ability to build the body's immune system. Coconut oil is now being recognized by the medical community as a powerful tool against immune-system diseases.

In summary, here is a list of cooking oil options:

Best
Olive oil
Sesame oil
Canola oil
Soybean oil
Coconut oil
Ghee and butter

Not as Good
Safflower oil
Sunflower oil
Corn oil
Peanut oil

By referring back to these lists, you will be better prepared to apply the different dietary suggestions of the Mars and Venus Diet and Exercise Program. Keep in mind that this program works because you don't have to use willpower and you shouldn't. The most important elements are drinking minerals, brief exercise, and the morning shake. You can then follow your natural desires and eat what you want and how much you want.

12

EATING FOR YOUR BODY TYPE

Practically everyone in America overeats and is unhealthy, yet only 65 percent of our population is overweight. Many of those overweight people eat much less than the lean or more muscular members of the population. An understanding of blood sugar and our different body types can help us to understand why some people eat the same junk food but are not overweight.

**Most overweight people eat much less than
the lean or more muscular members of
the population.**

The lean members of our population also eat too many nutrient-deficient carbohydrates (or fats and proteins). They are driven by desires for unhealthy food. When their blood sugar rises and more insulin is produced, the excess energy is processed differently. Instead of being stored as extra fat, the energy is utilized by the muscles or the brain. The brain burns calories just as the muscles do.

Instead of gaining weight, some people use up this extra energy through addictions or through worrying and obsessing. When your brain or muscles are overstimulated, you will burn more calories. For some people, overthinking will burn excess blood sugar, while others burn extra energy by being overly active. Your body type determines how you process high blood sugar levels. There are basically three body types:

1. The round type. These people are born with more fat cells. This number of fat cells does not change in a lifetime. Becoming overweight means these fat cells expand. Men and women of the round type are round at the belly, like an apple. If they have a poor diet, they will commonly suffer from weight gain. Spending too much time in a gym or overexercising actually inhibits fat burning in their bodies.

2. The triangular type. Triangular women have an hourglass shape, and triangular men tend to be more solid and square, with a tapered waist. Triangular types are born with more muscles than the other body types. If they have a poor diet, they will tend to overexercise or become addicted to something. If they don't exercise, they too will get fat. These people easily lose weight just by increasing their exercise schedule.

3. The rectangular type. Both men and women of this type tend to be long and thin. If women carry extra weight, it tends to be in their hips and thighs. If men carry weight, it is generally in the belly. They are rarely overweight, and excess weight is primarily the result of toxins stored in the body. These persons tend to be lighter with smaller bones. Under stress, they will often lose their appetite, but when blood sugar drops, they will crave unhealthy food and have a huge meal. They have thin bodies and tend to suffer more from increased anxiety and compulsive disorders. The extra energy for high blood sugar is literally used up by the brain, causing it to become overactive.

Under stress, thin people will often lose their
appetite for a while and later overeat.

Regardless of body types, there can be other health factors that contribute to weight gain or loss. Medications, missing organs, concussions, genetic defects, and an imbalance in particular glands can also affect weight gain. Most commonly, an imbalanced thyroid gland can cause any body type to gain or lose weight.

By far the most significant factor influencing weight and mood management is the food we eat. The poor diet that we eat often activates genetic sickness or an imbalance of hormones produced by the glandular system. The body is incredibly adaptable and resourceful when given the right balance of foods and an opportunity to cleanse itself of accumulated toxins.

Keep in mind that no one is ever a pure body type. We always have a combination of at least two types. One is dominant and one is secondary. William Sheldon conducted a tremendous amount of body type research in the 1940s. For our purposes, this research helps explain why men and women have their own unique requirements for a healthy balance of dietary fat, protein, and carbohydrates.

In summary, excess sugar in the blood caused by an imbalanced diet is processed in three different ways:

1. Excess fat storage is a round person's reaction to high blood sugar.
2. Exercise addiction or hyperactivity is the muscular person's most common reaction to high blood sugar.
3. Excessive brain activity—worry and anxiety, for example—is the lean person's reaction to high blood sugar.

No person is purely one type, and each of us has a unique combination of all three body types, and suffers to various degrees the symptoms of all three reactions to imbalances in blood sugar.

Before exploring in greater detail how we can eat for our particular body type, let's first understand why we commonly eat the wrong foods.

WHY WE EAT THE WRONG FOODS

People with low blood sugar can eat a high-sugar snack or a meal packed with refined and processed foods, and feel better immediately. Of course they will continue to want those foods that give them an immediate reward. All their bodies know is that they were starving and suddenly felt better. This benefit is false because one or two hours later, they will crash back down, feeling low energy again.

This is not the only reason we crave unhealthy foods, but it explains a big part of the problem. Other reasons include low production of brain chemicals, mineral deficiency, enzyme deficiency, and different degrees of malnutrition or nutritional deficiency. Let's do another quick review of the relationship between insulin and low blood sugar for those who are not fully familiar with these ideas. Considering that Americans eat a pound of sugar each month, we cannot hear this explanation enough. Maybe this time, it will sink in.

INSULIN AND LOW BLOOD SUGAR

When you eat processed foods or refined carbohydrates (sugar, white bread, cereals, pastries), the sugar from these foods gives your body quick energy. The food goes into your stomach, and sugar is quickly released into the bloodstream to feed your muscles and brain. If you were eating enough fiber, minerals, protein, and fat with these carbohydrates, the sugar would be released in a slower, healthier fashion. It would go to the liver first, and be released in a closely regulated fashion to maintain stable blood sugar levels.

In a high glycemic carbohydrate snack that is deficient in nutrients, such as a bag of chips or some cookies, the sugar is released so quickly into the blood that the body has to release insulin from the pancreas to lower the sugar level. Too much or not enough blood sugar affects brain functioning in a negative manner. If the carbohydrates you ate were filled with minerals and balanced with protein and good fats, your blood sugar level would remain balanced.

When blood sugar is low, we crave nutrient-deficient carbohydrate food to raise blood sugar for energy.

The big problem with releasing insulin to lower blood sugar is that we tax the pancreas. After a while it produces too much insulin. Think about baseball. When the pitcher is fresh, he can throw strikes right over the plate. When he is tired, he loses his accuracy. When the pancreas ages and is tired of producing emergency insulin to lower the blood sugar, it becomes less accurate. When blood sugar rises, too much insulin is released, lowering the blood sugar too much. As a result, your energy level drops way down. This drop can happen very suddenly, particularly in women. If they don't get some quick energy, they will become very cranky.

To lower the blood sugar level, the hormone insulin converts the excess sugar in the blood to be stored in the muscles and liver. Any extra is stored as body fat. The blood sugar levels drop again. At this point, we crave more fast energy foods to raise blood sugar levels. Once again, more insulin is required to lower the blood sugar and store the excess energy. With another wave of low energy, we begin to crave more nutritionally deficient food for fast energy. This explains why we keep craving unhealthy food. There is a false benefit of energy to a starving brain, but it is short-lived and then we crave more food again.

Now we are ready to add to this information the understanding of our three body types and how our dietary needs and vulnerabilities are different according to the body type with which we were born.

UNDERSTANDING THE THREE BODY TYPES

Let's explore in a little more detail the different dietary requirements for people with different body types. Dr. Sheldon labeled them endomorphs, mesomorphs, and ectomorphs:

• **Endomorphs** (round shape) are characterized by a high percentage of body fat, a relatively small amount of muscle mass, large bone size, and slow metabolism. These people may have a more difficult time in athletics, and will have a harder time achieving desired results in the gym, particularly if they attempt to be model-thin.

• **Mesomorphs** (triangular shape) typically possess a large amount of muscle mass, a low body fat percentage, medium to large bone size, and a rather high metabolism. Mesomorphs are suited for sports that require good strength and short bursts of energy. They must be careful not to become addicted. Even with addictions to healthy behaviors like work or exercise, they will have less brain power and may need to sleep too much. Too much exercise can also lead to accelerated aging.

• **Ectomorphs** tend to make good endurance athletes. They have a slight and youthful appearance and possess a low body fat percentage, small bone size, and a high metabolism with little muscle mass. They generally have little interest in working out in a gym, as they are too busy living in their minds and dreams. Although they typically don't have excess weight, with accumulated toxins they may have weight gain around the waist as they get older.

1. THE ROUND BODY TYPE

More fatty acids (not less!) from good dietary fat are required for the round type. This recommended increased level of fat required for the round type is still much lower than what is considered to be a low-fat diet in America. In comparison to the other two types, the round person needs a little more fat, but in comparison to our national average, which is 100 to 200 grams a day, a round person needs much less fat. According to U.S. dietary guidelines, we only need between 70 and 80 grams of fat a day.

All women would benefit from a low-fat breakfast supplement adding a full tablespoon of fresh flaxseed oil (13 grams of fat) or, even better, 2 tablespoons of freshly ground flaxseeds (11.4 grams of fat). Men will benefit from a third to half a tablespoon (approximately 7 grams of fat) or, even better, 1 tablespoon of freshly ground flaxseeds (5.7 grams of fat). If you are overweight, you definitely need more good fats to start burning your stored fat. Good fats are essential for burning body fat, building healthy tissues, and, most important, regulating the production and balance of our hormones.

Eating good fats burns body fat.

Experts claim that the maximum any body can actually ever use in a meal is around 15 to 25 grams of good fat. Many obese women eat well over 75 grams of fat in a meal, but their bodies are actually starving for good fats. Round types need to make sure they eat three meals and at least two small but balanced snacks a day. A balanced snack means a little protein, carbohydrates, and fat. A few nuts and raisins is a good example; nuts have balanced protein and fat, while raisins provide the carbohydrates.

One reason obese women put on so much weight is that they eat too much bad fat and not enough good fat. Their cells are literally starving for more fat to burn the excess fat. They will tend to crave "low-fat" junk food filled with trans fats or bad fats.

Without a proper balance of good omega-3 and omega-6 fatty acids, all women, round or not, suffer unnecessarily. The average person in America has an extreme deficiency of omega-3 fatty acids. With an omega-3 fat deficiency, women commonly experience PMS as well as uncomfortable menopause symptoms. For both men and women, a host of deadly diseases, from cancer and arthritis to heart disease, have been linked to too many bad fats and a deficiency of omega-3 good fats. For all body types, a supplement of omega-3 in the morning is the secret to healthy hormone production and balance.

Eating too much bad or good fat causes some weight gain for round types, but eating high glycemic foods is the most common culprit. We usually eat more quick-burning carbs (pastries, cookies, desserts, and sugar in our coffee) to raise our blood sugar to get the energy our brains need. Eating food to raise blood sugar for the round type is like earning more money than you need. What do you do when you have too much money in your checking account? I hope you put it in your savings account to earn interest or put it in a safe investment. Well, this is what your body does. When there is too much sugar in the blood, it converts that sugar into stored body fat for a time of need.

That extra fat sits there waiting for you until you need it. As long as excess insulin keeps getting produced, fat just keeps accumulating instead of being burned as fuel. This means you keep getting fatter and fatter, craving more and more fats and carbohydrates.

**Excess insulin blocks the conversion
of excess fat into energy.**

For your body, rising and falling blood sugar is similar to living through a time of an unstable stock market. If every day the stock market is going way up and way down, many investors keep their extra money in a secure retirement fund. In a similar manner, until your diet supports steady blood sugar, your body will store fat.

When you have adequate fatty acids and proteins in your diet to slow down the release of blood sugar, insulin levels become normal and your excess fat starts to burn off your body.

If you have excess weight, starting your day with a low-calorie, nutritionally dense breakfast gives your body all the energy it needs for hours. Right away, your body starts burning the excess fat, and you feel as though you have boundless energy!

2. THE TRIANGULAR BODY TYPE

More amino acids from a well-balanced protein diet are required for the muscular type. An adequate supply of protein, while maintaining a healthy number of calories, can be difficult to achieve for all types. Most meat and other animal products today have a much lower than ideal ratio of protein to fat. Farming practices, including hormone injections and grain feeding instead of free-range grass feeding, have changed the balance of protein to fat in farm animals.

An animal today is sold based on weight. As a result, most farmers do whatever they can to increase the body fat of their animals. What they do to fatten up their livestock and chickens will fatten you up as well. Not only is there too much fat in the meat we eat, but the balance of good fats has changed. Instead of being a somewhat equal balance of omega-3 to omega-6 fatty acids, there is now ten to twenty times too much omega-6. Although the fats are good fats, there is an imbalance of fatty acids.

This means our chicken, beef, and turkey servings all have too much omega-6 good fat and not enough omega-3 good fat. To solve this problem, always go for free-range animal products. When selecting your proteins, always go for lean cuts so that you don't get too much fat. Fish has an excellent balance of protein to fat. Salmon, mackerel, cod, and tuna are high in omega-3 fat and have the best balance. By supplementing your diet with high-protein, low-fat foods or with protein powder, you can be assured of not getting too much fat, which can inhibit the processing of amino acids into brain chemicals.

Fish have an excellent balance of protein to fat.

Triangular bodies use up protein more quickly than other types because of their muscles. If all the protein is consumed, there is not enough left for the production of dopamine in the brain. Triangular bodies need a higher balance of protein to fat.

Too much fat or carbohydrate will cause an insulin response, which sends all the amino acids to the muscles, leaving none for the production of dopamine. Recent research reveals a link between excess fat and high blood sugar. Excess fat inhibits glucose utilization by the muscles, resulting in high blood sugar, which then leads to an insulin response. Men's bodies, rectangular bodies, and muscular bodies are more vulnerable to this reaction. With fewer fat cells, a man needs less fat. For all body types, a balanced protein mix in the morning activated by minerals and enzymes to produce healthy brain hormones is the secret to proper brain balance.

Too much fat or carbohydrate will inhibit the production of dopamine.

Being more muscular, triangular types and all men require more exercise. This is why men can generally lose weight faster than women. They have more muscle mass, and the mitochondria in the muscle cells burn fat very efficiently. Mitochondria are contained within a cell. They are responsible for burning calories by breaking down food molecules and releasing the energy inside. Most of our mitochondria are located in the muscle cells. To burn excess body fat, muscles need to be used or exercised. To build muscle, they need to be exhausted, they don't need to be injured. Sedentary triangular types will put on extra fat if they don't keep their metabolism at a normal level by using their muscles. If they don't exercise, their metabolic rate slows down, and they begin to store fat and become overweight. Exercise is essential, but too much exercise is not desirable.

Without enough exercise, the metabolic rate slows and we begin to store fat and become overweight.

What is too much exercise? Running for seven miles for most people is too much, even though it may make them feel high as a kite. I have too many friends who at fifty need knee surgery from jogging. The golden rule for everyone is, If your exercise gets you out of breath or causes you to feel sore afterwards, you are doing too much.

A little moaning and groaning in the gym is great, but if you are not enjoying every bit of it, then it is too much. Even if you enjoy it, if you are sore the next day, you are damaging your body and inhibiting the proper production of brain chemicals. You will also know you are exercising too much if you feel tired or bored at other times.

The triangular type tends to overexercise because too much exercise produces a high from endorphins in the brain. This is a false benefit, because overexercising uses up the amino acids in the blood and blocks the continuous production of dopamine in the brain, which is associated with a man's energy and intelligence levels.

Too much exercise blocks dopamine production.

With intense exercise, all the amino acids go to the muscles, and none are left to produce the feel-good brain hormone dopamine. In addition, all the blood sugar is metabolized and little is left for the brain. The brain gets all its energy from carbohydrates. When these are gone, there is nothing left for the brain.

Overexercising is particularly harmful for students. It is no coincidence that athletic types in school often have difficulty keeping their grades up. The jock is a stereotype, though body type, just like gender, has nothing to do with intelligence. But overexercising can make you less focused, less motivated, and less attentive. Too much exercise will lower dopamine levels and decrease the activity of the prefrontal cortex in the brain.

It is no coincidence that athletic types in school often have difficulty keeping their grades up.

We have previously discussed that the prefrontal cortex of the brain determines attention span, judgment, impulse control, problem solving, critical thinking, the ability to feel and express emotions, communication, and empathy—basically all our higher executive functions. Without enough dopamine produced in the brain, it is no wonder that one in five boys in school are diagnosed with ADD or ADHD, or that 90 percent of the people in jail are men. Not just muscular types are particularly vulnerable to low dopamine, but all men and boys. Men generally have 20 percent more muscle than women, even triangular women. Though exercise is essential and more important for men than for women, overexercise is worse. It creates the symptoms of low dopamine in men, and inhibits fat burning in women's bodies.

Overexercise creates the symptoms of low dopamine in men and inhibits fat burning in women's bodies.

When women do intense or even moderately intense exercise, the mitochondria in muscle cells burn carbohydrates instead of fat. As a result, fat burning is inhibited. A woman will temporarily feel good but gain weight. Moderate and not intense exercise is best for women.

My favorite book on this subject is *The 24-Hour Turnaround* by Dr. Jay Williams. By providing a holistic anti-aging approach for women's health and weight management, she explains in great detail how different forms of intense exercise can literally sabotage a woman's efforts.

Women often work so hard to keep weight off and care for their bodies, but without the right Venusian-friendly exercise, it is all for nothing! In her program on the Big Island of Hawaii, Dr. Williams has proven with thousands of men and women that in just twenty-four hours, you can feed and exercise your body, mind, and spirit to achieve a complete turnaround.

We have taught many workshops together, and I have personally experienced why many celebrities, entertainers, and corporate executives who can afford the best personal trainers seek out her expertise. She emphasizes that what you do and eat each day determines how you will feel. What you have done yesterday is much less important than what you do today. Healing and growth is a one-day-at-a-time process.

With proper diet and exercise, you can begin producing the right brain chemistry in twenty-four hours.

Men tend to be low in dopamine and intense exercise lowers it even more. As a result, muscular men tend to have more problems with addiction and ADD and ADHD symptoms. With the exception of overeating and smoking, most addictions are symptoms of low dopamine. Overeating and smoking for women is generally a symptom of low serotonin, *not* low dopamine. We have already explored in Chapter 3 how addictive stimulations help a man to compensate for lower levels of dopamine in the brain.

Most addictions—except overeating and smoking— are symptoms of low dopamine.

Triangular vegetarians need to be careful with their protein consumption. To supply all the essential amino acids required to produce brain chemicals, vegetarian sources of protein must be combined. Grains, vegetables, legumes, nuts, and seeds all have plenty of proteins, but on their own they don't form a complete protein. Animal proteins—fish, meat, poultry, eggs, and milk products—already have a complete balance of all the essential amino acids. With a wide variety of foods, vegetarians can easily get the protein they need.

In India, where vegetarians are common, one of the staples of the diet is lentils and rice. These two foods combine to produce a complete protein. In Mexico, the common combination of rice and beans provides all the essential amino acids. In Asia, soy products are commonly eaten. The soybean provides all of the essential amino acids. Soy is a miracle replacement for those who choose not to eat meat. Each day, more and more benefits are reported from the use of high quality soy products. Hemp (which is not the same as marijuana) is the only other nonanimal protein that has all the essential amino acids. It is a yet-to-be-discovered miraculous source of protein. It also has the ideal ratio of omega-3 and omega-6 fatty acids.

The soybean provides all of the essential amino acids.

Vegetarians are frequently deficient in vitamin B_{12} according to published studies. Fermented soy products (tempeh) and seaweed or vitamin supplements are the only known nonanimal sources of B_{12}. Without enough B_{12} we become depressed. B_{12} is required for the conversion of amino acids into dopamine and serotonin.

Vitamin B_{12} is required for the conversion of amino acids into dopamine and serotonin.

When blood sugar rises, muscular people can use up this extra energy by overexercising. If they have an injury and can't overexercise, their muscle turns to fat. By overexercising the muscles, they enjoy the pleasure of increased endorphins in the brain at the expense of unnecessary wear and tear to the body, which speeds up the aging process.

After a big workout, many bodybuilders experience extreme fatigue and sleep a lot. Not only does their blood sugar drop, but this sleep is the result of deficient dopamine in the brain. The extra sleep is always required by the body, because the muscles need to rebuild, which occurs during sleep. When they get more sleep, their brains can replenish depleted dopamine levels.

3. THE RECTANGULAR BODY TYPE

The rectangular person requires more sugar (or glucose) from good carbohydrates. Everyone, regardless of body type, needs plenty of carbohydrates. Generally speaking, 50 percent of our calories need to come from good carbs. It is the sugar from carbs that feeds our brains and nourishes our cells. Sugar gives us energy and alertness. Fat is also burned as fuel for energy, but the brain, which uses the most energy, can get its energy only from carbohydrates. Fatigue is linked to low blood sugar. Staying alive, awake, aware, and enthusiastic—all this comes from healthy blood sugar levels.

The brain can get energy only from carbohydrates.

The brain really doesn't care what kind of carbohydrates you eat. All carbs break down into sugar, and that is what the brain wants and needs. Without sugar we die. Oxygen and water are more important than sugar, but sugar is next on the list of important nutrients. No one in America has a problem getting enough carbohydrates and sugar. Our widespread problem is too much sugar.

People with a lean body type tend to use up the extra energy of high blood sugar with excess brain activity. In short, they think or feel too much. When blood sugar surges, their brains begin to use up this excess energy. As a result, rectangular types can become overly analytical, anxious, emotional, or obsessive-compulsive. Thin people suffer most from brain imbalances. By eating more complex carbohydrates like grains and legumes, they will have a steady flow of energy. Too many simple carbohydrates (sugars) will increase symptoms of brain imbalance.

Thin people suffer most from brain imbalance.

From this perspective, people who show their imbalance in blood sugar by having weight problems can see that they are sick and that their diet is causing premature aging. The muscular and athletic types, who are working out all day in the gym or who jog seven miles a day, think they are healthy because they look so good. Then suddenly some of them drop dead from a heart attack. The joggers are all having knee surgeries at fifty. The skinny folk, who can eat whatever they want and don't require exercise to stay thin, are busy worrying about other things and have no idea that their diet may be killing them as well. They think it is just genetics that is causing all their ailments.

**Lean people eat whatever they want
without weight gain and think
genetics is causing all their ailments.**

Rectangular types tend to be sugar-sensitive. They experience mood swings. They crave high glycemic foods for quick sugar, and then their blood sugar drops along with their energy and mood. This means that they easily get caught up in carbohydrate hell.

The symptoms of high and low blood sugar include feeling cranky, distressed, tired, hungry, confused, weak, and shaky. Millions of men and women are plagued by these symptoms of chronic low blood sugar. They may seek out counselors for help when what they are really missing is a healthy, balanced breakfast. One of the first things that occurs in the Mars and Venus Solution is a natural balancing of blood sugar. Without a need for junk foods, you will find a stability for yourself and your children that many just can't imagine. The shift occurs in days.

Mineral supplementation is essential to reduce sugar cravings and stabilize our blood sugar levels. A deficiency in chromium causes excessive sugar and high glycemic food cravings. Chromium is commonly found in soil in most regions of the world. Until recent times, people obtained chromium by eating foods with natural concentrations derived from the soil. Today our lands are depleted of trace minerals.

CHROMIUM DEFICIENCY

For the past century, modern agriculture has relied on chemical additives like seasonal replenishment of nitrogen, potassium, and phosphorus. The result is high crop yields every year in which these three basic farm fertilizers are replenished. Over the years, the other naturally occurring essential minerals and trace elements, including chromium, have been farmed out of the soil and not replenished. Thus, most of our foods are chromium-deficient at the level of agricultural production. As our food has become deficient of chromium, our sugar consumption has continued to rise.

In his brilliant book *Achieving Vibrance,* Gay Hendricks points out that one hundred years ago, Americans ate about a pound of sugar a year. We used sugar only for special occasions and used it in small doses, a spoonful a week. Now, he points out, the average American eats more than a hundred pounds of refined sugar a year. Nearly everything you can buy in a can, box, or package off the shelf has refined sugars, refined fats, or refined flour to give us a quick high, only to be followed by a mental fog twenty minutes after eating. *Refined* means all the other nutrients like minerals and fiber have been removed. This imbalance wreaks havoc on our bodies.

The average American eats more than a hundred pounds of refined sugar a year.

Food processing further reduces chromium (and other essential minerals for human health) by as much as 90 percent. The result is widespread nutritional chromium deficiency, compounded by lifestyles that further compromise chromium levels. Chromium deficiency can result in anxiety, fatigue, loss of mental clarity, vision impairment, reduced immune response, unwanted weight gain, acne, glucose-intolerant conditions (hypoglycemia, diabetes), unhealthy cholesterol levels, and plaque buildup on the arteries.

Researchers have known for decades that people who died of heart disease had abnormally low chromium levels. A recent study shows that patients with heart disease have as much as 40 percent less chromium than is found in the blood of people enjoying cardiovascular health.

People who die of heart disease have abnormally low chromium levels.

Chromium's importance in proper health and vitality is based upon its cofactor role as a regulator of insulin. When a person is deficient in chromium, insulin does not function properly, which in turn can result in potentially dangerous levels of blood sugar.

If our food was not chromium-deficient, dietary chromium could be found in whole grain cereals, brown rice, broccoli, meat products, cheeses, dairy products, eggs, mushrooms, peanuts, and potatoes. Chromium is also found in such herbs as thyme, cinnamon, catnip, licorice, and in pepper. All kinds of peppers—black, chili, cayenne, and bell—are high in chromium. Kava is also a member of the pepper family and is well-known for its ability to stabilize blood sugar and particularly encourage the production of serotonin. Since chromium is not fully available in our food today, chromium supplementation is essential to sustain your blood sugar levels.

Chromium supplementation can break the cycle of overeating sweets. Eating sweets causes chromium deficiency, while simultaneously causing drastic increases in insulin and glucose levels. Chromium deficiency can trigger a person's craving for fattening sweets, which causes the cycle to repeat. When insulin is functioning efficiently, blood sugar and fatty acids metabolize properly, producing heat (thermogenesis) instead of weight gain. Research suggests that weight loss diets achieve improvements in body fat burning as a result of dietary chromium supplementation.

Chromium deficiency can trigger a person's
craving for fattening sweets.

Bodybuilders have taken chromium supplements for years because of the mineral's vital role in protein metabolism and converting body fat to muscle mass. Some sports nutritionists believe that chromium slightly increases muscle mass even without exercise, perhaps as a result of improved insulin sensitivity. Chromium supplements have been shown by researchers to be effective in the treatment of acne as well. Chromium supplementation is required every day as an integral part of the Mars and Venus Solution.

DR. ATKINS' DIET REVOLUTION

Dr. Robert C. Atkins first popularized the low-carb diet in 1972 in his convincing book *Diet Revolution*. He provided the perfect balance for the once popular Pritikin diet, which recommended a *high*-carb, low-protein, and low-fat diet. The American public went from one extreme to the other. This was an important and healthy move for many. An extremely low-fat diet is not healthy, but neither is an extremely low-carb diet. More and more experts are agreeing that balance is the solution.

The main reason some people feel great on Dr. Atkins' low-carb diet is that eating more proteins and fats makes it easier for them to stop eating the bad carbs, like processed grains and refined sugars. After a few days on a high-protein, high-fat diet, many people stop suffering from carbohydrate cravings and are released from blood sugar hell. This can be a tremendous relief for all body types, but particularly for the rectangular type.

After a few days on a high-protein and
high-fat diet, many people are released from
blood sugar hell.

Dr. Atkins' popular diet, which has been attacked by many experts, may be good for some people if they strictly follow the rules and don't overeat protein and fats. He does mention a maintenance diet in which you eat more and more vegetables, which are good carbohydrates. The problem with this diet is that some people don't follow it strictly and eat way too much meat or bad fats, which is not healthy. Without an abundance of complex carbohydrates, the brain doesn't get fed. The brain needs plenty of carbohydrates to function. Without enough carbohydrates, women are the first to fall off the diet due to serotonin-induced food cravings.

If your car is overheated, it is good to turn it off and let it cool down. This, however, doesn't solve the problem. You have to add water to the radiator before you can run the engine without it overheating. A low-carbohydrate diet can lower insulin levels for sugar addicts, but it deprives the brain of the glucose it needs. Cutting out all carbohydrates is as extreme as giving a mental patient a lobotomy, like cutting out parts of the brain if they are overactive. There are certainly better ways to relax the brain than simply turning it off by cutting off its fuel supply. In his new book *Atkins for Life,* Dr. Atkins addresses the importance of incorporating good carbohydrates in his maintenance program.

Research continues to show that high-protein, high-fat dietary patterns, when followed over the long term, are associated with increased risk of degenerative diseases. Here are the most important:

1. Cancer. Long-term high intake of meat, particularly red meat, is associated with significantly increased risk of colorectal cancer. Keep in mind that this red meat is not free-range meat, which is leaner and has more omega-3 fats. In addition, high-protein diets are typically low in dietary fiber. Fiber facilitates the movement of wastes from the digestive tract and promotes a biochemical environment within the colon that is protective against all disease.

2. Cardiovascular disease. Typical high-protein diets are extremely high in bad fats. A recent study showed that the consumption of a high-fat meal (ham-and-cheese sandwich, whole milk, and ice cream) definitely contributed to heart disease.

3. Kidney stones. The American Academy of Family Physicians notes that high animal protein intake is largely responsible for the high prevalence of kidney stones in the United States and other developed countries, and recommends protein restriction.

4. Osteoporosis. Elevated protein intake is known to encourage urinary calcium losses and has been shown to increase the risk of fractures. When carbohydrate is limited, this calcium loss is magnified.

The temporary beneficial effect of low-carbohydrate diets for reducing insulin levels are real, but risking the known side effects is not worth it, since there are other ways to keep blood sugar balanced.

THE MYTHS ABOUT LOW-CARB DIETS

There is a lot of misunderstanding about the benefits of a high-protein, high-fat, and low-carbohydrate diet. Let's explore a few common myths:

1. High-protein diets cause dramatic weight loss. The weight loss typically occurring with high-protein diets is approximately 20 pounds over the course of six months. This is not any different from what has been observed with other weight-reduction regimens involving low-fat or vegetarian diets. The high-protein and high-fat diet is popular because eating more fats makes it easier to give up bad carbs.

2. Fatty foods must not be fattening. Some people mistakenly assume that because Americans are supposedly eating a low-fat diet yet are getting fatter and fatter, a low-fat diet doesn't work. This is not true. Americans are eating more fat and sugar. Food surveys from the National Center for Health Statistics from 1980 to 1991 show that the daily per capita fat intake did not drop during that period. For adults, fat intake averaged 81 grams in 1980 and rose to 86 grams in 1991.

3. People who eat the most carbohydrates tend to gain the most weight. This belief is completely wrong because rectangular body types eat the most carbohydrates, and they often have no problem with weight. For round people, processed and refined carbohydrates turn to stored body fat. This has been misinterpreted as suggesting that carbohydrate-rich foods are the cause of obesity.

In studies and clinical trials, the reverse has been shown to be true. Many people throughout Asia consume large amounts of carbohydrate in the form of rice, noodles, and vegetables, and they generally have lower body weights than Americans. Vegetarians, who generally follow diets rich in complex carbohydrates, typically have significantly lower body weights than nonvegetarians.

EAT MORE AND WEIGH LESS

In his book *Eat More, Weigh Less,* Dr. Dean Ornish clearly points out the many health dangers of a high-protein diet as well as pointing out the many benefits of his low *bad* fat diet. Dr. Ornish recommends a low-fat, plant-based diet that uses fruits, vegetables, whole grains, beans, and soy products in their natural forms. This incorporates moderate quantities of egg whites and nonfat dairy or soy products, and small amounts of sugar and white flour. These foods give you a double benefit: They are low in substances that are harmful, and are rich in hundreds of substances that may be protective against heart disease and many other illnesses. With this diet, you can eat as much as you could ever want and lose weight as well. He also dispels the myth that you have to eat less to lose weight.

This program is often criticized for being too low in fat for the average healthy person. The only other problem I can see with his program is that, unless you are very motivated, it is hard to follow. Many people with heart disease have turned to Dr. Ornish's program to reverse the disease. It is so effective that many insurance plans cover this program for symptoms of heart disease and prevention. If you are relatively healthy and very busy, it might be hard to find the motivation to follow all the requirements.

The Mars and Venus Solution added to Dr. Ornish's program could make it even more effective. With the balance of brain chemistry that results from following *The Mars and Venus Diet and Exercise Solution* in the morning, one can easily be motivated to stay on a healthy diet program like the one he suggests.

THE DANGERS OF SUGAR

The weight loss benefits of Dr. Atkins' low-carb diet are also similar to the short-term benefits achieved for the people who read and followed the immensely popular book *Sugar Busters*. Probably the best thing Americans can do for their diet is to stop eating so much refined sugar. Without a doubt, anyone who makes this change will begin to lose weight and feel better. For that, I am most thankful for the success of *Sugar Busters*.

At the same time, I was suprised when diet drinks and sugar replacements containing aspartame were recommended instead. There is a controversy concerning aspartame, particularly active on the Internet. Some sources contend that aspartame is not harmful; others hold that aspartame may cause dangerous side effects, especially when it is heated. I come down on the side of caution and do not recommend aspartame as an alternative to sugar.

The truth is that there are some very safe, sane alternatives to sugar, but the food services industry has failed to pick up on these. Stevia, an herb five hundred times sweeter than sugar, has been shown in studies to stabilize blood sugar levels over time and, in some cases, even to reverse some of the damage of diabetes. It's been in use in Europe for centuries, and has no known adverse side effects.

Stevia, an herb five hundred times sweeter than
sugar, has been shown in studies to stabilize
blood sugar levels.

The best alternative to sugar is simply to cut back on it. When you eat a sugar-rich dessert, another antidote is to take a really good trace mineral supplement in a glass of water with lemon. Minerals and lemons are known to reduce your blood sugar by 30 percent. In addition, drinking minerals will alleviate the necessity of leaching minerals from the bones to process the sugar. Another problem with refined sugar is that it changes the pH of your body and makes it more acidic. A little dose of lemon to taste will help restore your body's healthy alkaline pH.

13

YOUR BODY IS DESIGNED
TO HEAL ITSELF

The body can heal itself when we provide it with the necessary support. Besides good nutrition and exercise, one of the ways we can help the body is to lessen our dependence on coffee, tea, and alcohol.

For the Mars and Venus Diet and Exercise Program to work, you do not have to give up stimulants right away. It is actually best to start the program for a week just to set the routine. If you drink coffee or tea to get going in the morning or drink beer and alcohol to relax at the end of the day, take a week before giving up your daily dependence on them. By starting the program, you will be laying the foundation to eventually release all dependence on drugs, alcohol, and stimulants.

Once you have set up the routine for the week, start giving up your bad habits. Each time you give up a bad habit, your liver first has to clean house, and your sense of dependency will be gone. When the toxins are gone, you will be free from another addiction or craving.

Eventually when your weight is normalized and you are addiction-free, then it is fine to drink coffee, tea, or alcohol now and then, and to enjoy occasional junk food if you wish. I am not dependent on these things for my well-being, but sometimes they are just fun and I enjoy them.

When you have a clean liver, it is fine for most
people to drink a moderate amount of coffee,
tea, and alcohol.

To manage my own weight, I first ate a very healthy Mars and Venus diet. In a few weeks I lost fifteen pounds. After stabilizing my weight, I could relax and occasionally eat junk and treats without negative effect. Always remember, to benefit from this program, you don't have to have a perfect diet or be perfect!

Perfection is not a requirement for experiencing
health, happiness, and lasting romance.

If you return to being dependent on bad habits, you can always stop again. This time, it will be easier because your liver will be much healthier, and you will have the support of balanced brain chemistry. It is much easier to change a habit once you begin producing adequate amounts of dopamine and serotonin.

CHANGING YOUR UNHEALTHY HABITS

Most people automatically stop feeling the craving for caffeine products after applying the Mars and Venus Solution. Giving up smoking is a little more difficult. Research shows that giving up smoking dramatically lowers serotonin levels. Lower serotonin levels have a much more devastating effect on women than on most men. Alcohol and coffee addiction stimulate the production of dopamine. That is why these are the most difficult addictions for most men to overcome.

In either case, after a few weeks of the Mars and Venus Solution, changing your unhealthy habits will become much easier. Once you have set up an easy and healthy routine, you will become more motivated to care for your body and brain in a healthy way. If you still feel controlled by addictive cravings after a few months of being on this program, rather than continuing to struggle, intravenous amino acid supplementation may be the easy answer for you.

Of the 51 million Americans who smoke, 90 percent say they want to stop but just can't. This is because smoking temporarily raises serotonin levels, and giving it up significantly lowers them. Even men, who have significantly higher levels of serotonin than women, become dependent on the cigarette to produce needed levels of brain chemicals. After a few weeks on this serotonin-producing diet, you will find it significantly easier to kick the habit and begin breathing fresh air again.

Of the 51 million Americans who smoke, 90 percent say they want to stop but just can't.

With this new understanding of the importance of brain balance to change our habits, we can all take a more compassionate position when we consider those who are afflicted with addictions. Millions of people are literally powerless to make a positive change in their lives. Even with psychological counseling and all the TV programs that say, "Just say no," many people cannot change unless they first begin to balance their brain chemistry.

WHAT HAPPENS WHEN YOU CHANGE A BAD HABIT

As soon as you give up an unhealthy habit, two things occur that appear to sabotage your efforts to feel good and healthy. The first is a reduction in brain neurotransmitters or feel-good hormones. This imbalance can lead you to crave stimulants again. If you are already following a brain-balancing diet and exercise program, this reaction is not felt at all or is very mild.

The second reaction to giving up any unhealthy stimulant like too much eating, too much alcohol, too much coffee, or too much sugar is that as soon as you make the change, your body decides to get rid of toxins. Your liver says, "Oh, great, you are not overworking me with all these toxins. Now I can start cleaning house."

As soon as these toxins get released into the bloodstream your mood and energy level may drop, unless you are getting proper amino acid supplementation, and you will seek out your stimulant or bad habit to feel good again. With *The Mars and Venus Diet and Exercise Solution,* you now know how to help your liver clean house every morning when you wake up. Without stimulants or drugs, you will be directly feeding your brain what it needs to feel good.

After making a positive change, toxins
get released, and it is more difficult to
sustain the change.

Giving up an addiction generally takes about nine days of willpower and amino acid supplementation, and then the addiction is gone. When fed healthy food, the brain takes about nine days to get back in business. Even with the right diet and exercise, it can take longer if your liver is severely weakened from a lifetime of drinking and taking drugs.

As soon as you change a bad habit, the liver begins to remove all the stored-up toxins that were caused by the addictions. During this time, the liver can be so busy detoxifying that it doesn't have an adequate opportunity to assist in the synthesis of necessary neurotransmitters. Depending on the condition of your liver, it may take more time to experience the dramatic results others experience immediately. One of the complications associated with drug and alcohol addictions is that they weaken the liver. The Mars and Venus Solution is designed to strengthen your liver so that it can most effectively do what it is designed to do.

TREATING SICKNESS AT THE CAUSE

The Mars and Venus Diet and Exercise Solution will give your body the support to do what it is designed to do. Though the program will not heal your health issues, it will help your body to heal itself. Your body is designed to be healthy. When it is diseased, through accidents, poisoning, and exposure to stress, it is designed to cleanse itself of toxins and heal itself of sickness.

Western medicine is best at treating symptoms, but it is only now just catching on to treating sickness at the cause. Holistic, preventative, and complementary medicine are becoming increasingly common as more doctors realize that people want more than quick fixes and symptomatic relief. Modern science, like a teenager who thinks he or she knows everything, is now maturing into an understanding that there is much more to healing than prescribing drugs, radiating cells, and removing organs.

People today want more than symptomatic relief; they are seeking natural ways to stimulate lasting healing.

A variety of doctors and medical facilities have included such other systems of healing in their treatments as chiropractors, naturopathic doctors and nutritionists, homeopathy, traditional Chinese medicine, intravenous ozone therapy (legal in Germany but not yet in the United States), prolo therapy, intravenous amino acid supplementation, vitamin supplements, acupuncture, herbs, aromatherapy, energy healing, spiritual healing, chi kung, tai chi, yoga, meditation, massage, positive visualization, and journaling.

A variety of doctors and medical facilities have included other systems of healing in their treatments.

Each of these different healing modalities stimulates the body's ability to heal itself in a variety of ways. *The Mars and Venus Diet and Exercise Solution* does not replace the need for this kind of healing support. The Mars and Venus Program only enhances the benefits of these healing modalities by giving your body the fuel it needs. Diet and exercise provide the oil and gas for the car. Benefiting from your doctor or healer is like taking your car in for a checkup or repair. We will always need the assistance of these different programs. With the Mars and Venus Solution, these programs will all work better and you will not need them as often.

Diet is like filling up your tank, and healing
treatments are like taking your car in for a repair
or regular service.

In my experience, all these systems work. They are great, but they work so much better when you supplement your day with extra nutrients and exercise. There are many books that document the value of these different treatments, so I will only explore a few that are most relevant to brain chemistry.

AMINO ACID SUPPLEMENTATION

For getting off any and all addictions, amino acid supplementation is a powerful and efficient treatment. In many cases, providing intravenous supplementation of missing amino acids can eradicate the symptoms of ADD, ADHD, autism, anxiety, manic depression, schizophrenia, and substance abuse of all kinds within nine days. If you supplement the brain with amino acids, the body can begin to produce healthy brain chemistry. When the starving brain is fed what it needs, it can begin to function normally, sometimes for the first time.

I have witnessed people go off their addictions without experiencing withdrawal symptoms. As we have learned, people only become addicted because they are deficient in dopamine or serotonin. When healthy brain chemistry is manufactured, all the addictive cravings just go away. The need for an addictive substance is replaced by the healthy need for dopamine- and serotonin-producing foods. By applying the Mars and Venus Solution, these patients have the ideal follow-up program to sustain these miraculous results and live free of their addictions.

There are more clinics for this kind of treatment opening up each day. I often recommend that people visit Dr. William Hitt's clinic, because I know they are getting these results. Soon I will be opening a Mars and Venus resort and alternative healing facility and spa on Little Exuma, an island in the Bahamas. People will be able to get these treatments while enjoying a relaxing vacation in the Bahamas. Those treatments are now available at the William Hitt Center in Tijuana, Mexico.

HOMEOPATHY FOR BRAIN TRAUMA

Homeopathy is recognized in Europe as a viable medical treatment, but is not yet widely practiced in America. Holistic doctors are generally trained in aspects of it and respect its principles. This medical treatment does not have side effects as pharmaceuticals do. You may have seen a variety of homeopathic remedies for different ailments in your health food store. These remedies stimulate the body's healing abilities. The practice of homeopathy is two hundred years old and has been well documented. Although many American researchers don't yet fully understand how it works, the results have been researched around the world.

The practice of homeopathy is two hundred years old, and the miraculous results have been well documented.

Homeopathy is particularly helpful for creating the brain chemistry of health, happiness, and lasting romance. It includes an effective treatment designed to stimulate healing in the brain. This treatment particularly interests me, because a small percentage of people who start the Mars and Venus Solution don't get the dramatic results that almost everyone else gets right away. The reason for this is that either they have a very toxic liver, which cannot yet produce adequate neurotransmitters, or they have experienced some trauma to the brain.

If you have a toxic liver, it may take several months before you get dramatic results. If in your past you have experienced some trauma to the brain, homeopathy can help dramatically. Trauma to the head does not necessarily mean a permanent disability. Brain trauma is like a broken bone. When a bone is broken, it will become whole again and be stronger than before if it is put in a cast to rest for a couple of months. The doctor resets the bone and puts it in a cast, and then nature does the rest.

Brain trauma is a similar situation. You bang your head and the pituitary gland gets shocked. The pituitary gland, located at the base of the skull, is the master gland that regulates all of the brain's other glands. When it is altered or adversely affected, it may cause a range of problems throughout the body, and in the brain itself. Unless something is done to stimulate healing in this gland, your ability to produce healthy brain chemistry may be restricted for the rest of your life. Many people have survived accidents, but their brains have not. Accidents and injuries, regardless of how long ago they occurred, can be the source of chronic physical, mental, and emotional disorders. With effective physical therapy treatments, bones may have healed, but a person may remain depressed or anxious. Instead of treating the trauma in the brain, they are given antidepressant drugs. For the rest of their lives, they go from one drug to another seeking temporary relief.

So many people have survived accidents, but their brains have not.

Injuries to the brain are more commonly known as brain concussions, and may result from womb traumas, difficult births, car accidents, falls, or sporting activities. Immediately after a brain concussion, headaches and dizziness may occur.

These symptoms can last for a period of time and then disappear. What is not commonly realized is that after the disappearance of the early acute symptoms, the patient is left with long-term, often subtle chronic problems. Some symptoms may not manifest themselves until many years after the traumatic incident.

Western medicine is great for resetting broken bones, but it does very little for concussions. Brain concussions are very common. They occur all the time, particularly for children at play and in sports. After small accidents, your brain can generally heal itself if you are eating enough minerals. If we don't get enough minerals in our diet, the brain's ability to bounce back and heal itself after a concussion is limited.

After a car accident, our bodies heal, but not always our brains. The brain is very delicate. It is the most protected organ in the body. If the skull is shocked or cracked, it can have lasting effects. Many people who were completely normal before an accident begin to suffer from all kinds of depression and panic attacks. Without direct treatments for brain trauma, people spend a lot of money and the rest of their lives in counseling or on prescribed drugs. Sometimes, in a matter of a few weeks, all the symptoms of brain trauma are gone after a simple six-week homeopathic treatment.

Taking mineral supplements years later will certainly help, but it may not be enough. Homeopathy has a very effective treatment for brain concussions that can speed up this healing. One small or large brain concussion left untreated can cause depression, anxiety, or erratic moods for a lifetime. Even very slight brain trauma that goes untreated can affect a child's whole disposition and continue into his or her adult life.

A concussion left untreated can cause depression, anxiety, or erratic moods for a lifetime.

I have been very impressed with the results of homeopathy for healing brain concussions quickly and effectively. I have had the treatment, and it worked wonders for me. I fell out of a tree headfirst when I was a second grader and broke both arms. My arms healed, but nothing was done to heal my concussion. That injury caused all kinds of problems during my life, particularly in times of stress. From headaches to mood swings, I had them all. This simple six-week treatment was able to correct the residue of this old wound.

This treatment is inexpensive and can be administered by parents to their children. It is completely safe, and there are no side effects.

The need for this treatment is even greater today. We don't have enough nutritional support to bounce back effectively from accidents and traumas. Most people don't realize that they may have had many different traumas to the body and the head. Traumas to the body can also cause trauma to the brain.

It may be that you have suffered a trauma to your body and brain, and it is affecting your ability to sustain a positive mood, lose weight, or think more clearly. Take a moment to remember your past. See what memories come up when you are asked these questions:

- Think back to a time when you went to a hospital. What happened?
- Did you fall out of a tree and break an arm?
- Did you ever hit your head, chin, or forehead on something so that it swelled up like a golf ball?
- Did you fall off a bicycle at some time and hurt yourself?
- Were you ever in a car accident?
- Did you ever get hit from behind?
- Were you ever dropped as a baby or did you hear stories of your falling out of bed?
- Did you hit your head on the bottom or side of a swimming pool or diving board?
- Did you ever get hit in the face with a ball, and it hurt?
- Were you ever hit and knocked down?
- Did you ever have the air knocked out of you?

- Did you fall down hard while skating or skiing?
- Did your mother experience an extra-long labor when you were born?

If you answered yes to any of these questions, you may have suffered a little brain damage that has never quite healed. One of the side effects of growing older is that all of our weaknesses are magnified if we are nutritionally deficient.

If you consistently hurt your wrist falling down as a young skater, you may have not noticed any problems. But later on, as you get old and your body begins to ache, it is your wrist that hurts the most.

The stress of nutritional deficiency always shows up first in our weakest or most wounded areas.

A few years ago, I had an accident that pulled my thumb completely backwards. It quickly went back into the socket, but it was very painful and never quite healed. When I started taking regular doses of omega-3 oil, the pain went away within three days. Now I am completely free of pain. If I occasionally don't get enough oil in my diet, I notice the symptoms of fat deficiency as I once again begin to feel pain in my stiff thumb joint, my barometer. When I am deficient in nutrients, it first shows up in my weakest areas. When I treat my body with what it needs, my thumb stops feeling stiff or painful.

Any blow to the head can shock the pituitary gland for the rest of your life unless it gets a little support to heal. Even blows to the body can shock the pituitary gland, although it is not as common or devastating. The older we get, the more we are actually affected by these old wounds.

As we get older, we can be increasingly affected by the wounds of childhood.

A hundred years ago, homeopathy was more effective because the food we ate had more minerals. Today, homeopathy is less effective unless it is complemented with mineral and enzyme supplements. If after a month of applying the Mars and Venus Solution you don't get the results you are looking for, you may need to look into getting a homeopathic treatment for brain concussion. One of the main symptoms of brain concussion, even if it occurred fifty years before, is the inhibition of balanced brain chemicals. With the insights of the Mars and Venus Diet and Exercise Program, along with the amazing potential of homeopathy, you can now help your body overcome any past traumas.

To understand more about homeopathic treatments for brain chemistry, you can visit www.homeopathicwonders.com, or call Dr. Salar Farahmand in Encino, California, at 818-501-2000 for a consultation. Dr. Farahmand is a world-renowned expert in the treatment of brain trauma and has developed a simple but effective treatment you can do at home.

AROMATHERAPY

One of the easiest ways to accelerate and sustain the benefits of *The Mars and Venus Diet and Exercise Solution* is with aromatherapy. Research has shown that the mind associates certain experiences with certain smells. If you wear a healing and uplifting essential oil fragrance, your brain will begin to link the production of serotonin and dopamine with this smell. After this link is made, just by application of the essential oil of your choice, you will find that your brain is stimulated to produce more healthy brain chemicals during the day.

Using essential oils is a potent healing alternative for almost every ailment, and particularly helpful for the brain. Thousands of people have been able to replace the need for prescription drugs with aromatherapy. At stressful times in our home, my wife will use essential oils in a diffuser to fill the air with peace and healing.

> Thousands of people have been able to
> replace the need for prescription drugs
> with aromatherapy.

Just as healing herbs all have special properties of healing, so do different aromatic smells. Essential oils are the fragrant, subtle, volatile liquids extracted by distillation from plants, shrubs, flowers, trees, leaves, roots, bushes, and seeds. These oils contained in nature have the regenerating, oxygenating, and immune defense properties of plants. When we expose our bodies to these essential oils, they serve as a catalyst in delivering oxygen and nutrients to the tissues of the body.

> Increasing oxygen to the brain stimulates the
> production of healthy brain chemicals.

Without oxygen molecules, nutrients cannot be fully assimilated, and the disease process begins. All brain dysfunction is associated with a nutritional deficiency of oxygen. Not only do essential oils contain oxygenating molecules, they also have a bioelectrical frequency. Frequency is a measurable rate of electrical energy that is constant between two points. Clinical research shows that essential oils have the highest frequencies and may create an environment in which disease, bacteria, virus, and fungus cannot live. My favorite essential oil is rose oil. It happens to have the highest frequency. In my experience, smelling and wearing rose essence directly stimulates the production of healthy brain chemicals.

Essential oils were mankind's first medicine. Egyptian hieroglyphics and Chinese manuscripts indicate that priests and physicians were using essential oils thousands of years before the time of Christ. There are 188 references to oils in the Bible. We have all heard the story of the Three Wise Men bearing gifts to the newborn Christ Child. They brought the oils of frankincense and myrrh. Clinical research has now found that frankincense oil contains very high properties for stimulating the immune system.

The Three Wise Men bearing gifts to the newborn Christ Child brought the oils of frankincense and myrrh.

Science is only now rediscovering the healing substances found in essential oils. You can find high quality essential oils at your health food store, and read all about their healing properties in a variety of books. To receive their amazing benefits, you can wear essential oils, massage parts of your body with them, or diffuse them in the air. My wife and I use high quality Living Young Essential Oils.

WHAT DOES YOUR DOCTOR KNOW?

If you are currently under the supervision of a doctor, you of course need to talk with him or her before applying any of the ideas in this book. Keep in mind that many medical doctors have only received a few hours of training on nutrition in medical school, and they are often too busy to keep up with all the recent research about diet and nutrition.

Many medical doctors and psychiatrists have received only a few hours of training on nutrition.

Doctors are faced every day with suffering patients on the one hand, and drug sales representatives touting the benefits of the latest new wonder drug on the other. It is hard to say no to drugs, when the people you care for are suffering and what you have already offered is not working.

In asking for your doctor's supervision, inquire about how many hours of nutritional training he or she has received. Keep in mind a naturopathic doctor receives at least four years of nutritional training. If your doctor's training in nutrition doesn't seem adequate to you, it is probably a good idea to seek a second opinion. Today there are many more holistic doctors and alternative health experts who are trained in nutrition as well as other forms of complementary healing modalities.

Let me give you two dramatic examples to illustrate this point.

DOES DIET AFFECT YOUR HEALTH?

Three years ago, Carol attended a three-month healing workshop I was teaching for people with life-threatening sickness. These people needed a lot more than *The Mars and Venus Diet and Exercise Solution*. We met three times a week, practicing together the self-healing techniques I teach in my book *Practical Miracles for Mars and Venus*. Carol was one of twenty-five participants who had stage 3 or stage 4 cancer. During the first couple of weeks, three participants died. They were literally too sick to do the techniques at home or even come to all the meetings.

Before coming to the workshop, most of the participants were expected to die within a couple of months. Everyone in the program, even those who eventually died, reported that they received tremendous emotional benefit and spiritual uplift from the self-healing techniques I was teaching. Within the three-month period, fifteen participants experienced complete remission from all cancer symptoms. This was miraculous. Their doctors were completely amazed, as were the members of their families.

Within a three-month period, fifteen participants experienced complete remission from all cancer symptoms.

Two more died, but family members came and told us how much the group had helped their deceased loved one through this difficult time. The other five participants stayed the same or improved, but at least they didn't get worse, as their doctors had predicted.

Carol was one of the group who eventually experienced full remission, or what some call spontaneous healing. During the first week, after being instructed in some of the dietary changes required for the program, she asked her doctor about them. His response was shocking.

He told her that it didn't matter what she ate. He then backed up his prescription with the comment that "There is no research to indicate that improving your diet could help you heal this cancer. Just enjoy eating whatever you want."

This message is very common. Besides being inaccurate, it is very misleading and dangerous. One of the most important principles of the Mars and Venus Diet and Exercise Program is that a healthy body wants healthy food, and an unhealthy body wants unhealthy food. When you are sick, you need more, not less, guidance regarding what to eat. If you are unhealthy, you cannot eat just what you want, because what you want will be unhealthy. By learning to start your day with a healthy breakfast, you will not only set your metabolism to burn the food you eat throughout your day, but it will set you up to want healthy foods and set you free from unhealthy cravings for sugars, stimulants, and bad fats that kill.

When we are sick, we need more, not less, guidance regarding what to eat.

A healthy body can endure a little junk food, but a nutritionally deficient person with cancer or any other life-threatening disease needs to eat with the same precision as a doctor administering drugs. If you eat too much of the wrong foods, your body's natural ability to heal itself is severely compromised.

A healthy body can endure a little junk food, but
a severely sick person cannot.

If a doctor told me that nutrition didn't affect my body's capacity to heal cancer, I know that I would quickly be looking for another opinion. With this information about food and how it affects your health, happiness, and love life, you will possess an important tool you have been missing. As you put this program into practice, you will learn that what you eat and how much you eat is the single most important factor for both physical and mental health.

WHAT DO YOU EAT FOR BREAKFAST?

My second example comes up regularly from callers on my radio show and in the questions at my seminars. Callers will ask, "Are you saying that I can start this program and give up taking my antidepressant?"

My answer is always the same. When you are under a physician's care, it is important that you consult with your doctor, communicating the changes you are making in your diet to lessen and eventually eliminate your dependency on drugs. Under a doctor's supervision, gradually diminish the amount of drugs you are taking.

The caller will then inevitably ask, "Do you think if I follow this program, I can be depression-free *and* drug-free?"

My response is: Before I can answer that question, let me ask you another question. Did your doctor who prescribed Prozac to you or Ritalin to your child even ask you, "What do you eat for breakfast?" Did they first put you on a healthy diet and exercise routine to see if that lessened or eliminated your depression?

Every time, the answer is "No, they didn't ask me about my breakfast, nor did they prescribe a specific diet or exercise routine."

With all the new research available about nutrition and depression, it is a tragedy that drugs are still prescribed without even a basic exploration into a patient's diet. If a person is indeed brain-damaged or experiencing dramatic psychological symptoms, then prescribing psychoactive drugs along with counseling can temporarily have a lifesaving and miraculous effect. If there is no emergency, it is best to first understand a person's diet and exercise routine. By suggesting and then observing the benefits of healthy alternatives, a trained professional can more accurately determine if a person really needs drugs.

The prescription of any drug has serious consequences and should not be taken lightly.

For some people, the option for a lifetime of prescription drugs is a miracle blessing from modern medicine. If a patient is just nutritionally deprived, as I believe most people are who are medicated, then a prescription drug is like a jail sentence. For the rest of your life, you are forced to live with the shackles of its side effects.

Most of the millions of people taking psychoactive drugs like Prozac are not mentally ill, but simply nutritionally deficient.

In the future, we will look back on this time with its widespread use of prescription drugs and shudder, as we now do when we look back just a hundred years and consider the medical techniques involving draining a patient's blood or performing a lobotomy. Even with patients who do have brain damage, there is now a growing body of research available that supports the ability of amino acid supplementation and homeopathy to assist the body in healing itself so that drugs are not necessary in some cases.

Without a complete understanding of the principles that underlie *The Mars and Venus Diet and Exercise Solution,* both adults and children will continue to be overmedicated. There is a good reason for this oversight. The natural alternatives to drugs are not yet mainstream. Many of the insights in this book are based on research only published in the last few years. This research reveals the importance of certain amino acids to produce correct brain chemistry. The practical applications of this research, called activated amino acid supplementation, are not even known to most of the researchers.

I have been searching for this breakthrough since my younger brother, diagnosed with manic-depression, shot himself nearly twenty years ago. The side effects of his drug treatment were so uncomfortable that he could not bear to live anymore. When he died, I committed myself to finding a natural cure for mental illness without requiring drugs and their debilitating side effects.

DEPRESSION-FREE WITHOUT DRUGS

Most doctors are not fully aware that there may be a danger in going off prescription drugs. Some believe that a rare side effect of commonly prescribed antidepressants or ADHD drugs is violence to others or violence to yourself.

The withdrawal symptoms of street drugs are a primary cause of the street and domestic violence we see rampant in our society today. Similar symptoms may occur when patients with "legal" drug addictions begin to stop.

Although the side effects of taking psychoactive drugs are unpleasant for many, the withdrawal symptoms can be much worse. Some studies suggest as many as 85 percent of patients who take psychoactive drugs may experience some degree of withdrawal symptoms when they stop. These include flulike symptoms, nausea, electric shock sensations, nervousness, violent behavior, suicidal depression, and melancholy. These are some of the symptoms that motivate these people to take drugs in the first place.

When these old symptoms reappear, patients panic and start taking their drugs again. By applying *The Mars and Venus Diet and Exercise Solution,* you can greatly assist your body in restoring normal brain balance without these side effects, but it takes some time. Wise doctors recommend taking several weeks or even months to lessen the required drug dosage gradually. The longer you have taken the drug, the longer it takes to go off.

As long as you are taking drugs, the benefits of *The Mars and Venus Diet and Exercise Solution* will definitely be limited. You will be helping your body and brain, but it will be like swimming upstream instead of downstream with the current. Each day you will be giving your body what it needs to produce healthy brain chemicals with the Mars and Venus Solution, and by taking drugs, you will be telling your brain that there is enough serotonin and more doesn't need to be produced. In addition, you will be putting more toxins in your body instead of cleaning them out.

A study reported in *The Journal of Clinical Psychiatry* reports that 70 percent of general practitioners and 30 percent of psychiatrists do not know the side effects of ending serotonin-boosting drugs. Many professionals do not warn their patients that if they want to discontinue the drug, they must do so very slowly.

It takes time for the brain to adjust and to produce healthy and balanced levels of serotonin on its own. Before discontinuing the use of a drug with your doctor's supervision, assist your brain in producing the right chemistry on its own. By applying *The Mars and Venus Diet and Exercise Solution,* you will give your brain the help it needs to begin producing healthy brain chemistry without the usual withdrawal symptoms.

**Feed your brain what it needs
before going off drugs.**

Police officers know that the majority of crime occurs because of drug addicts seeking to get money for more drugs. After getting high and then coming down, they will steal and kill to get more. Most domestic violence is linked to illegal drugs, prescription drugs, or alcohol addiction. The withdrawal symptoms of going off a drug, either prescription or illegal, without some form of amino acid supplementation, are not only associated with intense suffering but are also dangerous to yourself and others.

Low serotonin is dangerous not only to ourselves but also to others. Research on male serial killers reveals brain dysfunction associated with extremely low levels of serotonin. When going off any drug, take time so that your brain can begin to produce serotonin on its own. Without a balanced diet and exercise routine, this may never happen.

When certain brain chemicals are low, addictions temporarily stimulate their production, and suddenly we begin to feel relief. When the brain becomes dependent on prescribed drugs, illegal street drugs, or any of our common addictions to stimulate the production of neurotransmitters, the brain thinks it is producing enough dopamine and serotonin. As a result, an already dopamine- or serotonin-deficient brain produces even less. When you stop using a drug or addiction to stimulate healthy brain chemicals, you may feel worse than before.

If you are currently addicted to something or taking a prescription drug, even with the right supplementation it will take a couple of weeks after you discontinue use to begin producing the necessary chemicals for normal mental health.

Before stopping drug use or attempting to change a bad habit, have in place a healthy diet and exercise program to fall back on. In addition, make sure that you are under the supervision of a trained medical professional. You can get a list of licensed medical doctors trained and experienced in the process of assisting people to go off prescription drugs at the Web site www.AlternativeMentalHealth.com.

There are also a few books that can help you. My two favorites are *Change Your Brain, Change Your Life* by Dr. Daniel G. Amen, and *Depression-Free for Life* by Dr. Gabriel Cousens. Every day these doctors and hundreds more like them help men and women heal their mental illness through natural means without always resorting to prescription drugs.

CREATING A WORLD OF HEALTH, HAPPINESS, AND LASTING ROMANCE

Ultimately, I believe that our global problems can and will be solved when men and women learn to share together to create a lifetime of romantic love. Why romantic love? Because romantic love is the first thing to go when our hearts begin to shut down in our relationships. Romance brings out the very best in men and women. And it is one of the most challenging goals. It requires us to grow in love, tolerance, forgiveness, and wisdom.

It is easy to get along if we bury our feelings. Staying in touch with the undying love in our hearts connects us to the highest part of ourselves. It tests and tempers us to be examples of what we all know is good and great. To experience lasting romance requires that we remain happy. If we are not happy, we cannot continue to feel the transformative fires of passion. They are always burning deep in our soul, but it is our challenge to awaken them again and again.

Taking responsibility for our happiness ultimately means finding the source of happiness within our hearts, a gift we are all given at birth but gradually lose. One of our challenges is to recapture that happiness. With the foundation of inner happiness, we mature into what we all can be: individuals fully capable of giving love without blaming others when we are not happy. If you want to blame something now, you can easily blame your biochemistry.

> **If you want to blame something now, you can easily blame your biochemistry.**

Staying happy to keep our hearts open is most easily achieved when you are healthy. By activating your body's healing power each day, you will grow in unconditional happiness. Perfection of life or health is not a prerequisite for happiness, but nurturing your body with what it needs to face your health challenges is.

As you do what is required to help your body heal itself or stay healthy, you will have the foundation for unconditional happiness, which then supports building the house of lasting romantic love. When there is no romance, people can still be wise, loving, kind, and compassionate, but not to as great a degree. Life without romance is devoid of the essence of love. It is more detached and reasonable, but it is missing the one element that can bring true and lasting peace in this world.

> **Life without romance is more detached and reasonable, but it is devoid of the essence of love.**

Romance can be sustained in a marriage only when we have learned to respect and appreciate our differences. This is a challenging task, but when we achieve this end, we are capable of meeting the greater challenges of settling disputes between the differences in our global cultures. It is too easy to put the blame on other countries, cultures, and their leaders, or our own, for that matter, when in our own lives we do not risk to open our hearts through forgiveness and sharing in the most intimate ways.

As the world becomes a smaller place, the need for better and more compassionate communication becomes a requirement. Many world leaders today persist in repeating the same behaviors that create the same problems. A solution to global tension and distress can and will be found as we the citizens of this global village are able to overcome the tension and distress in our own lives and in our own intimate village.

We cannot solve world problems while we are over-medicating ourselves. We must be able to face reality head on with clarity, wisdom, and compassion. We cannot solve the problems of the world when we can't keep our hearts open to our mates, children, family members, and neighbors. The battle is not out there. It is right here at home.

Peace in the world begins at home.

In all religions, the highest spiritual realization is the recognition that we are all one with nature and the universe. In this manner, we are all intimately connected. When you strive to overcome the challenges in your own life, you make it a little easier for everyone else to take the steps they need to take. When you take a step, you help everyone take a step.

When you strive to find love again rather than hold on to hate and resentment, you help the world open up more to love.

When you find forgiveness and let go of the past hurts in your life, the world forgives a little more.

When you practice living in present time and appreciating what you do have, you help the world move a little more into the present where problems can be solved, rather than dwell on the past, which we can do nothing to change.

This is a special time in which we live. We have the potential to enrich every aspect of our lives or blow ourselves up. The choice is ours.

We have the potential to enrich every aspect of our lives or blow ourselves up.

You have that choice when you begin creating healthy brain chemistry. When you neglect your body and brain, that choice is taken from you, and you are once again caught up in the petty concerns of overactive and underactive brains. You have so much more potential waiting to be actualized. Each step you take to achieve this end will not only help you but help the people you love.

For me, getting up to exercise and eating a healthy breakfast is not just for me but for my wife and family. I know that I am more loving and supportive when I do the right thing for my body and brain. I now know that my mind and body are intimately related. I also know that the way I treat my loved ones helps you and everyone else in this world. In some meaningful way, I make the difference every time I do what it takes to create the brain chemistry of health, happiness, and lasting romance.

I know that you will make this difference, too. Together, our efforts and our open hearts do make the difference. Thank you for sharing with me on this wonderful and exciting new adventure. I hope you share this with your friends and loved ones, as well. Please stay in touch and give me your feedback at www.MarsVenus.com. I am available to answer your questions and hear your comments and concerns. Most important, let me know your successes. It inspires me and everyone else who visits the Web site.

As you write and share your successes with *The Mars and Venus Diet and Exercise Solution,* it will become even more effective for you, for me, and for the others who also visit my Web site at www.MarsVenus.com. As you share this program, you affirm not only to others but to yourself that you can do it, and, most important, that you *are* doing it!

Share your success and your success will be greater.

Feel free to call me between 9 A.M. and noon, California time, while I am live on my radio show, and share your successes, questions, and challenges (1-888-MarsMan). If you wish to receive private coaching, I am not available, but you can get advice over the phone by calling the Mars and Venus Coaching Program (1-888-MarsVenus). These coaches have been trained to help you clearly identify your relationship issues, and then share with you suggested solutions from my thirteen Mars and Venus books.

Each weekday, you can hear me and my guests answering your questions about men, women, relationships, dating, parenting, health, diet, and exercise. The three-hour morning radio program is then recorded and replayed at www.MarsVenus.com at all hours of the day, on all days. With this support, let me assist you whenever I am available in whatever way I can.

With this support, you are not alone. If you choose it, I am there at any time. You have my support and I need your support. Together, we can make the difference for ourselves and the world. May you always grow in love and fully enjoy the benefits of creating the brain chemistry of health, happiness, and lasting romance.

Index

SPECIAL OFFER FOR YOU

Call 1-888-627-7836 for details on receiving
a free 10-minute coaching session.

Now you have the ability to talk with a MARS VENUS
expert when an issue comes up.
We all understand the power of information.
The more we know, the better we can deal with a situation.
No matter how successful we are, sometimes we all need to
talk about our problems to understand them better.

We have analyzed your most frequently asked questions
about relationships and have developed a coaching program
that not only provides information about the cause of
and solution to your problem, but also provides
a coach to guide you through your situation.

Call today for information about this service and you'll
receive a free 10-minute coaching session.

Your special pin number entitles you to one free 10-minute coaching session.

PIN = 527235

This pin number should only be used once.

Also, one caller per month will randomly be selected to speak to
John Gray personally for a free 20-minute session.

www.marsvenus.com

If you like what you have read, and you want more for your company, organization, or yourself, consider:

MARS VENUS IN THE WORKPLACE SEMINARS

Thousands of individuals and companies around the world have already benefited from John Gray's workplace seminars. We invite you to share an inspiring presentation or workshop with your company. MARS VENUS IN THE WORKPLACE seminars are designed to enhance gender communication in the workplace at all levels. Presentations are made by John Gray or one of his many trainers. Each seminar can easily be tailored to the unique needs of your company or organization. Please call our representatives toll-free at 1-888-MARSVENUS (1-888-627-7836) or visit John Gray's Web site at www.marsvenus.com for booking information.

ATTENDING A MARS VENUS WORKSHOP

The MARS VENUS INSTITUTE offers workshops that bring information to local communities and organizations around the world and trains those interested in presenting these workshops. MARS VENUS workshops focus on different topics, including improving communication, understanding differences, dating, starting over, parenting, and achieving personal success. These fun and insightful workshops feature favorite video segments from live seminars by John Gray, along with workbooks and exercises for participants to apply the information. A current schedule of workshops available throughout the world can be found on the Web site. To facilitate a workshop for your school, church, organization, or community, please call 1-888-MARSVENUS (1-888-627-7836). Becoming a facilitator is easy. You can be trained to present these workshops over the internet or through correspondence.

MARS VENUS COUNSELING CENTERS

In response to the thousands of requests we have received for licensed professionals who use the MARS VENUS principles in their practices, John Gray has provided a training program for licensed professionals to provide the MARS VENUS approach to their clients. Participants in this program have completed a rigorous study of John's work and have demonstrated a commitment to his valuable concepts. If you are interested in a referral to a counselor in your area or you seek information to be trained as a MARS VENUS counselor or to establish a MARS VENUS counseling center, please call 1-888-MARSVENUS (1-888-627-7836).

www.marsvenus.com

TALK TO A MARS VENUS RELATIONSHIP COACH

Reading John Gray's books and listening to his tapes have helped millions of individuals to improve communication and get what they want in their relationships. Whether you are single or married, it is never too late or too early to understand the ways men and women are different. This valuable resource can be enriched by talking to a MARS VENUS relationship coach on the phone.

When you feel the need to talk with someone like you or of the opposite sex, who is also familiar with the MARS VENUS principles and insights, he or she is only a phone call away. By calling a MARS VENUS coach you will receive personal attention to your specific needs. In the privacy of your own home, with complete anonymity, you can freely share your concerns and questions to sort out what you feel and then decide what you want to do. You decide when and how long you want to talk. Call 1-888-MARSVENUS (1-888-627-7836) or visit www.askmarsvenus.com.

EXPLORE THE WORLD OF JOHN GRAY AT MARSVENUS.COM

At www.marsvenus.com you will find information on the following subjects:

- John Gray's free weekly newsletter
- Workshops, seminars, coaching, and counseling
- John's weekly question-and-answer column
- The MARS VENUS Dating Site
- The MARS VENUS Store
- John's Calendar
- How to become a MARS VENUS facilitator, coach, or counselor
- Insight, advice, and shared experiences from all of John Gray's books and tapes, from personal relationships and parenting to achieving greater success at work

If you do not have internet access and would like the information on any of the above topics, please call toll-free 1-888-MARSVENUS (1-888-627-7836).

SHOP ONLINE AT THE MARS VENUS STORE

John's books, audio and video programs, and game are developed for all ages and stages of relationships. You can purchase all of his products easily online when you visit the store at www.marsvenus.com. Each week a different program is discounted specially for MARS VENUS online visitors.

If you don't have internet access and desire further explorations of the wonderful world of Mars and Venus, or if you wish to make an order or receive additional information, please call toll free 1-888-MARSVENUS (1-888-627-7836).

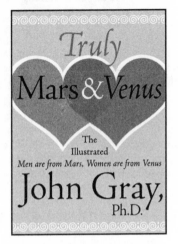

COUPLES' TRUE STORIES

MARS AND VENUS IN LOVE
Inspiring and Heartfelt Stories of Relationships That Work

Trade paperback 0-06-050578-8
Audio version read by the author:
2 audio cassettes / 3 hours (abridged) 0-694-51713-5

MEN ARE FROM MARS, WOMEN ARE FROM VENUS BOOK OF DAYS
365 Inspirations to Enrich Your Relationships

Hardcover 0-06-019277-1

KEEP PASSION ALIVE!

MARS AND VENUS IN THE BEDROOM
A Guide to Lasting Romance and Passion

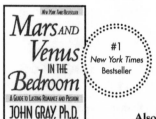

Trade paperback 0-06-092793-3
Audio versions read by the author:
2 cassettes / 2 hours (abridged) 1-55994-883-3
2 compact discs / 2 hours (abridged) 0-694-52215-5

Also available in Spanish: MARTE Y VENUS EN EL DORMITORIO
Trade paperback 0-06-095180-X
2 cassettes / 2 hours (abridged) 0-694-51676-7

MAKE LOVE LAST!

MEN, WOMEN AND RELATIONSHIPS
Making Peace with the Opposite Sex

Trade paperback 0-06-050786-1
Audio version read by the author:
1 cassette / 1.5 hours (abridged) 0-694-51534-5

MARS AND VENUS TOGETHER FOREVER
Relationship Skills for Lasting Love

Trade paperback 0-06-092661-9

Also available in Spanish: MARTE Y VENUS JUNTOS PARA SIEMPRE
Trade paperback 0-06-095236-9

A ROAD MAP TO DATING

MARS AND VENUS ON A DATE

A Guide for Navigating the 5 Stages of Dating to Create a Loving and Lasting Relationship

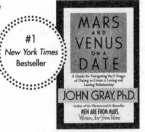

Trade paperback 0-06-093221-X
Audio version read by the author:
2 cassettes / 3 hours (abridged) 0-694-51845-X

OVERCOME LOSS & GAIN CONFIDENCE

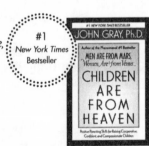

MARS AND VENUS STARTING OVER

A Practical Guide for Finding Love Again After a Painful Breakup, Divorce, or the Loss of a Loved One

Trade paperback 0-06-093027-6
Large print 0-06-093303-8
Audio version read by the author:
2 cassettes / 3 hours (abridged) 0-694-51976-6

BECAUSE PERSONAL DYNAMICS CAN MAKE THE DIFFERENCE

HOW TO GET WHAT YOU WANT AT WORK

A Practical Guide for Improving Communication and Getting Results

Paperback 0-06-095763-8
Hardcover (published under the title *Mars and Venus in the Workplace*) 0-06-019796-X
Audio versions read by the author:
6 cassettes / 9 hours (unabridged) 0-694-52655-X
2 cassettes / 2.5 hours (abridged) 0-694-52555-3
2 compact discs / 2.5 hours (abridged) 0-694-52560-X

MAKE PARENTING A POSITIVE EXPERIENCE

CHILDREN ARE FROM HEAVEN

Positive Parenting Skills for Raising Cooperative, Confident, and Compassionate Children

Trade paperback 0-06-093099-3
Audio versions read by the author:
2 cassettes / 2.5 hours (abridged) 0-694-52136-1
2 compact discs / 2.5 hours (abridged) 0-694-52170-1
7 cassettes (unabridged) 0-694-52163-9

www.marsvenus.com

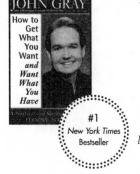

VIDEOS BY JOHN GRAY
JOHN GRAY TWO-PACK VHS VIDEOTAPE SERIES

In these five 2-pack VHS tape series, Dr. John Gray explains how differences between men and women—Martians and Venusians—can develop mutually fulfilling and loving relationships. Series includes:

MEN ARE FROM MARS, WOMEN ARE FROM VENUS
(2-Pack #1)
Tape #1: Improving Communication (60 mins.)
Tape #2: How to Motivate the Opposite Sex (56 mins.)

MARS AND VENUS IN THE BEDROOM
(2-Pack #2)
Tape #1: Great Sex (80 mins.)
Tape #2: The Secrets of Passion (47 mins.)

MARS AND VENUS TOGETHER FOREVER
Understanding the Cycles of Intimacy
(2-Pack #3)
Tape #1: Men Are Like Rubber Bands (45 mins.)
Tape #2: Women Are Like Waves (62 mins.)

MARS AND VENUS ON A DATE
(2-Pack #4)
Tape #1: Navigating the Five Stages of Dating (57 mins.)
Tape #2: The Secrets of Attraction (71 mins.)

MARS AND VENUS STARTING OVER
(2-Pack #5)
Tape #1: Finding Love Again (107 mins.)
Tape #2: The Gift of Healing (105 mins.)

For further exploration of the wonderful world of Mars and Venus, please call or write to place an order for additional information.

John Gray Seminars
20 Sunnyside Avenue #A-130
Mill Valley, CA 94941-1564
1-888-MARSVENUS (1-888-627-7836)

www.marsvenus.com

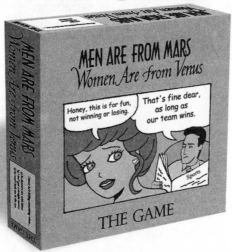